YOUTH:

Problems and Approaches

Edited by **S. J. Shamsie, M.D.**

Clinical Director, Thistletown Regional Centre, Rexdale, Ontario

Associate Professor, Department of Psychiatry, University of Toronto

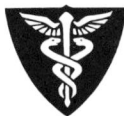

LEA & FEBIGER · 1972 · PHILADELPHIA

ISBN 0-8121-0404-8

Published in Great Britain by Henry Kimpton Publishers, London

Library of Congress Catalog Card Number 72-79353

Printed in the United States of America

PREFACE

This book represents an attempt to promote understanding and to provide some guidelines to those who are in a position to help the young. The number of people who are involved in helping youth is varied and large. Included in this group are not only professionals and parents, but also a large number of lay people working in youth clinics, hostels, juvenile courts, correctional institutions and a variety of other fields which have developed in recent years. There seems to be a clear need for a book that is not directed to professionals alone, but also aims to aid the many who are in a position to help the young. Such a book could also be a resource for the young themselves if they wished to use it.

After recognizing the need for such a book, I was faced with two questions: Is there a body of knowledge which is clear and precise? Can this knowledge be written in a manner which is simple and direct, so that it can be grasped by the many?

After discussion with a number of colleagues I was convinced that, although our knowledge may be imprecise, we have a body of considerable clinical experience which could be shared. I was also assured that professionals could be secured to relate their experiences in a language which would be largely free of technical terms. How far these hopes have been realized will have to be judged by the reader.

The book has three sections, each section opening with an interview. It was hoped that these interviews would present views in a more spontaneous manner and cover a larger field than would be possible by means of dissertations on specific subjects. An interview situation also allowed questioning the interviewees concerning some of their writings. In framing the questions the questioner tried to imagine what persons involved in helping the young would ask if they had the opportunity of talking with those interviewed.

I wish to express my thanks to Doctors Margaret Mead, Irene Josselyn and Maxwell Jones for agreeing to be interviewed. The interview with Dr. Margaret Mead was conducted by Dr. Unwin, and the other two by me. Dr. Unwin was very helpful in developing the framework of this book. He worked closely with me in the early stages and was generous with his time and advice.

I would also like to thank Mrs. Bederman who helped me in the editorial task and Dr. C. A. Roberts who made it possible by freeing her from other duties.

Rexdale, Ontario   *S. Jalal Shamsie*

ACKNOWLEDGMENTS

I gratefully acknowledge permission for publishing the following: "Developmental Psychology of Youth" by Daniel Offer, M.D., and Judith Offer in *Modern Perspectives in Adolescent Psychiatry,* edited by J. G. Howell, Brunner-Mazel Inc., New York. "Some Implications of the Sexual Revolution for Youth" by James F. Masterson Jr., M. D. This chapter will appear in Vol. II of *Adolescent Psychiatry,* edited by Sherman C. Feinstein and Peter Giovacchini, to be published by Basic Books Inc., New York. "Youth in Conflict" by S. J. Shamsie published in Laval Medical, Vol. 41, April, 1970.

S. J. S.

CONTRIBUTORS

William M. Easson, M.D.

Professor and Chairman, Department of Psychiatry, Medical College of Ohio at Toledo, Toledo, Ohio

Donald J. Holmes, M.D.

Consultant to Student Health Service Arizona State University and Arizona State Hospital.

Maxwell Jones, M.B, M.R.C.P.

Irene Josselyn, M.D.

Beryce W. MacLennan, Ph.D.

Acting Chief, Mental Health Study Centre, National Institute of Mental Health, Adelphi, Maryland

James F. Masterson, Jr., M.D.

*Professor of Clinical Psychiatry,
Cornell University Medical College,
New York, New York*

Margaret Mead, Ph.D.

Daniel Offer, M.D.

*Associate Director, Institute for Psychosomatic and
Psychiatric Research and Training,
Michael Reese Hospital,
Chicago, Illinois*

Judith Offer

*Research Associate, Institute for Psychosomatic and
Psychiatric Research and Training,
Michael Reese Hospital,
Chicago, Illinois*

Rix G. Rogers

*General Secretary, The National Council of
YMCAs of Canada, Toronto*

S. Jalal Shamsie, M.D.

Clinical Director, Thistletown Regional Centre,
Rexdale, Ontario
Associate Professor, Department of Psychiatry,
University of Toronto

John R. Unwin, M.D.

Director, Youth Services, Allan Memorial
Institute of Psychiatry
Associate Professor of Psychiatry, Faculty of
Medicine, McGill University
Montreal, Quebec

Rudolph Wittenberg, Ph.D.

Psychoanalyst in Private Practice
New York, New York

CONTENTS

Section III   Youth and Society

INTRODUCTION

Quentin Rae-Grant, M.D.

*Professor and Vice-Chairman, Department of
Psychiatry, University of Toronto*

*Psychiatrist-in-Chief, Hospital
for Sick Children, Toronto*

Youth, like sin, sex and taxes, has been from time immemorial a topic of angered, anguished and inconclusive
discussion. More recently it has moved into place of primacy in conversation, news media and publications as the
other subjects have declined in their value as detonators
of dissension.

Sin is now largely the province of the pedant, prelate
or primitive as the rest go about the job of doing it rather
than worrying or agonizing about it. Taxes rise so painfully
and persistently, that nothing and no one seems to stop
them and now little remains other than resignation to the
inevitable. Sex has been so subject to questionnaire,
interview, testing and photography that we now have all
the information while few of the facts about the people

attached to the frenetically busy genital apparatus. And the introduction of Kinsey, Ellis, Masters and Johnson into conversation is more likely to get the yawn rather than the blush.

But youth has maintained its heuristic value as a subject to stir the juices of controversy. While motherhood, apple pie and the flag have all bitten the dust it would be a rash fellow indeed who would brush aside youth, its problems and its anguish. For youth have collected all the violent feelings from the other topics. They are sinful. They don't worship the shower or soap or the obscenity of the military hair cut. They don't sit passively while teacher and professor bore them in a never ceasing drawl. They interrupt. They travel around. They beg without apology. They enjoy themselves, make a lot of noise about it even more when things are not to their liking. As to sex, they vigorously exercise their acclaimed principles of self-determination to make the sex manuals pale and unimaginative collections of platitudes. They even insist on doing and talking of this natural activity, naturally and with open honesty. Whether there is more activity than 20 to 30 years ago is questionable. There is certainly more talk and much more accusation against those who would, albeit now with trepidation, attempt a condemnation. The position has been reversed. The youth now have not only the physical vigor, but also the know-how and the opportunity. Maturity has nothing with which to assert its rights to control the young to compensate for lost chances or declining powers. It has only, as has always been true, envy, now unleavened by effective authority to forbid.

Further, there are simply more of them both in relative and in absolute terms. One-half the population of North America is under 25. And because of the post-war baby boom a large hunk of this lies in the youth area. They are also more affluent, both from their homes and from alternative sources now available. They have had the opportunity to be better educated and in some areas this is true though many have been so turned off by the fact of force feeding by the system that they junk anything and everything from the past or from others' experience. But they have effectively pushed us into concern with poverty and pollution and some way out of such tragic power trips as Vietnam. Certainly they are more vocal, less retiring, more challenging, less accepting, more experienced and experiencing and perhaps less content. They have demanded and received more political power, including the vote, and everyone runs scared as to what, if anything, they will do with it.

Thus, mention youth and zap! In one word you open a Pandora's box of those who do what we used to do or would like to have done, without guilt and with enjoyment and moreover do this on money from the ever-increasing taxes. Not only are they ungrateful, but even have the audacity to object to such things as the work ethic that holds the adults from time for these enjoyments, so that they can earn money on which to pay taxes to support these youth who accuse and mock them for a reward. Yes, youth is the present topic for discussion and embittered debate compounded and made more splutteringly angry by the fact that each individual has his own answers. Everyone, bar no one, feels he is a qualified expert on what adolescents are, what they should be and what they need, be it psychology, "sockology," social work or Siberia. Yet in this, as in so many areas of social science, the heat and conviction of the debate are in inverse proportion to the validated facts, which are even more difficult to obtain because of the wildly fluctuating nature of the youth scene. The knowledge will be gained slowly and erratically in small incremental accumulations with, of necessity, the modesty of each accumulation being an accepted expectation. Having created youth and adolescence as a prolonged transitional life period, we must develop an understanding of what we have wrought and keep in mind that the problems have been effected as much by us as by the youth and even more are amenable to changes through our actions. For change we must. We are all poorer by the degree to which any individual in our city, country or world is poor. We are all polluted by any pollution. But only we, individually and collectively, can change this, not the government, not business, not the U.N. or any group of "them" out there.

The youth have given us many lessons and, though they are the thorn in the flesh, so are they the conscience of the society. They have given fewer hostages to the system. They thus can show us, in a light we ought to have for ourselves, the inequities, the hypocrisies, the wasteful and ruthless ego trips that the system invites, encourages and rewards. They suggest ways for change short of the disaster of total revolution which would do no more than shuffle the ego trip opportunities. They have shown the trap of conspicuous consumption and, by example, demonstrated that the possession of innumerable appliances by the 20-year-old is no guarantee of happiness despite the commercial promise of life lysed of its difficulties. And they are experimenting with alternatives to the failure that is the nuclear family, though there are many questions as to the permanence of success for these alternative solutions. They have proclaimed that the city is for people and they have tried to inculcate a new series of personal worth values rather than position and possession status measurement.

As a conscience of the society they are probably more effective by numbers, involvement and persistence than at most times in history. But they or particularly their vocal leaders deliberately, it seems, handicap themselves by their anti-historical, anti-intellectual stance. Indeed their stance could well be labeled arrogant—arrogant to assume that all the questions and the answers can be derived from one's own head, arrogant to assume that no one else before has ever gone through these agonies of personal worth and meaning in life, arrogant to reject as of no value the previous answers tried, arrogant to dismiss previous very similar experiences, e.g. commune, kibbutz, monastic life, and, finally, hypocritically arrogant, while rejecting everything, to include those selected few philosophers who express theories that appeal often because they have the limited and limiting virtue of opposition. It is remotely tenable to dismiss everything of the past and of others as irrelevant to today but it then makes no honesty to tip the hat or bow the knee to the Marcuses, Reichs or Laings. He who demands honesty of others, must first require it of himself.

There are many mythologies of youth, about youth, and youth-adult relationships. The hackneyed concern over the generation gap assumes this exists, that it is undesirable and should somehow be bridged. It is assumed that the adult world is responsible for its existence. One must not omit to mention the breakdown in communication. Once again the patsy for this is the adult, square culture. Yet the processes of growth and development require privacy and independence and in some areas good communication is tantamount to maintained dependence, intrusion and timid sheltering. The adolescent does *not* need a constant circuit of communication but something more of a battery booster charge when periodically he dips into an available, accepting but not controlling, situation for renewed supplies of energy, hope and encouragement. If he tells all the question is who is going, through adolescence: this young person or the adult. Who then is helping and who exploiting whom? It is difficult for adults to trust their adolescents. They know it is a difficult period: they remember the awkwardness, the rebuffs and the very intense personal reactions to either success or rejection. They remember their own actions of both omission and commission. And they would willingly do anything to make the path easier for their kids. But they cannot and the knowledge that they cannot is frustrating, disappointing and alarming, particularly when their messages of caution seem often to be translated by their offspring into manuals of operation.

We know something of adolescents: we know the tasks of the stage: we have to learn the specifics from them as to time and place and practice. They are neither all good, pure, angelic and loving either to us or to themselves. But neither are they as revolted and revolting as some would have us see them. If we are to expect them to see us as individuals, we must do the same with them. The stereotype is easy to derive, safer to deal with than the individual who can affect and move us to love or hate. The stereotype draws its energy from our primitive being, depersonalizes us as individuals and leads us to condone wars, assassinations, brutality, repression, all of course for the good of those on whom these are inflicted. Stereotypes kill eventually both object and the person who initiates them. Many of our difficulties between youth and adult are between stereotypes, theirs and ours, both of them potentially or actually lethal. But both they and we are always surprised when we can talk and get beyond the image to the person and develop a sense of trust with those of different opinions, philosophy and values. If we can learn that to disagree about ideas or issues is by no means incompatible with respect and even warm friendship we may be able to help each other in collaboration rather than in a confrontation and conflict manner.

Our task is to admit how little we know, how much we must still learn, how tenuous are the methods we employ to help them and their families. Our task is not to retire in insult or hurt nor to embrace in unthinking enthusiasm every new (and often half-baked) idea that comes along. Our task is to be open, considerate and considering, both willing and eager to change. If we can accept change as the only constant of today, and we see the challenges and opportunity in it, we can then perhaps join hands rather than locking fists in a partnership for progress with the most valuable resource of a country— its young people.

SOCIOCULTURAL AND DEVELOPMENTAL ASPECTS

Chapter 1

YOUTH AND CULTURE: AN INTERVIEW WITH MARGARET MEAD

Dr. Mead's ground-breaking studies of communities in Samoa and New Guinea, in the late twenties, was the beginning of a remarkable career which has won the admiration and respect of all who are interested in understanding human behavior.

She lived for many years with South Seas peoples, learning their primitive languages and studying their customs. She observed how a child grew up through adolescence to adulthood. She studied the relationship between the young and the old and it is with this perspective gained by the study of small, homogeneous, stable societies that she looks at the present-day youth.

Dr. Mead in her interview looks at cultures hundreds of years apart and pinpoints similarities and differences in attitudes and ethics of the young. She explains how in many ways the young of today are different from any generation before, and how adults find it hard to accept this fact. With her understanding and empathy for the young, we see the present-day youth with hope rather than despair, with understanding rather than anger.

Question: Do you think psychiatry has tried to work with social sciences such as psychology, anthropology and sociology?

**Margaret
Mead:**   Well, modern psychiatry, clinical psychology and anthropology have been trying to work together to understand what has been happening. I do not think that one can make a general statement about psychiatry; there are places where there is considerable recognition of the cultural and social factors and then there are other places where there is not. In the past a lot of the assumed understanding between psychoanalysis or psychiatry and anthropology was a myth: anthropologists thought that they understood the super-ego and thought that it was the same thing as conscience, and psychoanalysts thought that they understood culture and that neither one of them understood what Freud had been talking about and so there was a magnificent degree of misunderstanding in both fields and I think to a degree it is still present.

Question: One of several reasons why we particularly wanted to interview you was that you have looked at quite a few cultures from the primitive to the western industrial and the the post-industrial societies and your initial work, of course, was very much concerned with youth (Mead 1928, 1939). One thing that fascinated me in reading *Coming of Age in Samoa,* which was published about 44 years ago, is the following passage which struck me as being quite contemporary. "The present problem of the sex experimentation of young people would be greatly simplified if it were conceived of as ex-

perimentation instead of as rebellion"
(Mead 1928). That could apply to today's
concerns that people have about the alleged
sexual revolution among young people.

Margaret Mead: Yes, except that we are still living in what I call a cofigurative culture. In my last book (Mead 1970) I have differentiated between postfigurative, cofigurative and prefigurative cultures.* In postfigurative cultures one could learn from the elders everything that there was to know, so that the child saw the end of things. In cofigurative cultures there is a reasonable amount of change so that each generation did have a change in style. In the 1920's in Canada and United States, where there were a large number of immigrants, young people had to learn from either other people who were here or set a style for themselves. As many of their parents had not been born here, the 1920's was very definitely a cofigurative culture when young people were learning from each other. In the prefigurative there are no adults to learn from at all, and many people think of this as rebellion, or alienation. The youth today do not want to follow the adult style as they consider it inappropriate to the modern world. They have no models so that they are experimenting and setting up their own style.

*Editor's Note: The following definitions are given in Dr. Mead's book *Culture and Commitment:* postfigurative culture, in which children learn primarily from their forebears; cofigurative, in which both children and adults learn from their peers; and prefigurative, in which adults learn also from their children.

Question: You have said, and I find it intriguing, that youth are the native born of the era and that the adults are first-generation immigrants. Could you elaborate on that?

Margaret Mead: Well you know, we were not born in the present modern world here, we were born under different skies, and, if we are going to pay attention to the modern world, it's a question of continually paying attention as an immigrant has to do. One can learn a new language, one can learn to live in a new country and one can learn a new style of life, but it is learned late as an adult and not learned as one grows up.

Question: This implies a need for radical reorientation of adults towards the era that they are living in, and towards youth, because I think the natural preconception of most adults is that it is their era and that the youth are the ones who are coming in as the immigrants.

Margaret Mead: That is right, it's a reversal of role, but we have always had it on this continent, this continent was founded, as far as Europe was concerned, by young adults, and when they woke up in the middle of the night they did not know what the different bird songs meant, and the children who grew up here did. On this continent, both in Canada and the United States, we have had a lot of experience of adult immigrants coming in and learning how to live here, so that we have a noisy type of superficial patriotism, because it is the patriotism of immigrants, not the natives.

Question: Do you sense any difference in the current politico-social climate between Canada and the United States, particularly in relation to young people?

Margaret Mead: Canada has always been more conservative. When our youngsters started getting married in college there was very little of that in Canada. Canada is more frugal; they have been operating on a much tighter budget educationally than the United States. In Canada young people were grateful for an education whereas in the United States they feel imprisoned in secondary schools and imprisoned in colleges. There is no sense of privilege whatsoever. If one starts with the immigrants, and one takes Canadian Italian immigrants and American Italian immigrants, the Canadian ones would be rather pleased if the third generation goes to the University and the children themselves would feel that they are privileged, that it will give them better jobs and a better place in society and so forth. But our third generation simply feel that they've got to go to college or they cannot get a job. This is the way it is being phrased in the United States.

Question: The belief that one does not get anywhere without a college degree, this sense of compulsion, is this what you mean by imprisonment?

Margaret Mead: The secondary schools are turning into a real prison. No student is allowed out of the building without a pass and in New York City one is not allowed out of a room without a pass; the teacher's main job is seeing that children do not get out of rooms without passes. In California they have towns where the police are looking around for young people who might be out of school. This is like a curfew; it is the same sort of thing as a curfew—any person who is on the streets is arrested—or as they treat Africans in South Africa. So the youngsters feel imprisoned. The education is vastly irrelevant; education has always been irrelevant to a degree, but if everybody believed that learning Latin turned you into a priest or a gentleman or whatever, then it did turn you into a priest or a gentleman because that is what the whole society agreed on. It was true of the Chinese classics and it was true of the schools in Eastern Europe. Learning to read Hebrew from dirty, torn, old books in a cold room where the teacher beat you with a cat-o'-nine-tails and berated you with obscenities was the way. They would say that the love of learning was born there and it was. Learning set you free, because then you could argue with elders and express aggression and grow up and it did not matter what learning was supposed to be, but that this turned you into what you wanted to be and there it was. But the minute you have teachers who cannot teach the way they were taught because the children they are teaching are too different, then the whole system breaks down.

Question: This brings us back to the concept of the current youth being the true natives and people talking about the generation gap. Would you say that it is more like an era gap than generation gap?

Margaret Mead: It is an era gap. I used the phrase "generation gap" as a subtitle for my book, which dates it, but I want it read now. I am not interested in books or articles being read as classics, but to get people to realize that the senior citizens of the new generation are now 24 and 25. This is very interesting because they are no longer youth, they are no longer rebellious college students, or wild-eyed high-school students, but they are getting into law, medicine and teaching. The youngest teachers are all in this era now and the adults are beginning to take them much more seriously. The adults are still screaming about long-haired kids in colleges, but they listen to the 25-year-olds, so that this is where the shift is going to come. I think that they will probably go right on vituperating the kids for quite a while and they will not notice what is happening, that we are having more and more parents who are listening to their children, because the children are now young adults and they are working.

Question: Now thinking in these terms, how does one persuade adults, and by adults I mean particularly professionals working with youth, to lay aside the more conventional pre-World War II concept of youth and reexamine, reconceptualize contemporary youth?

Margaret Mead: I think that there are two things here, they are living in fairly rapid change, but they are living on a very deep changed base. If you look at people before World War II, the older people moved from horses to automobiles and from candles and lamps to electric lights. The young never saw the candle, they have never lived in the world without the bomb, they never lived in a world where a major war would not destroy everybody. The people thought one could win wars and we did win World War II, for what it was worth, but we won it; we wanted to destroy Hitler and we did it; but today winning a war is impossible. The young live in this world; they have never lived in a world without TV. They have no sense of history; they're like pepole in the middle of New Guinea, who for the first time see a European. The New Guinean sees somebody who is completely clothed—he never had seen anybody with clothes. The European has a watch on his wrist, he has a flashlight, he has a ball-point pen, he has a transistor radio—objects that are hundreds of years apart in date of invention, but the native observer does not know this.

Question: Is this not also the immediacy, the shared experience that kids no longer learn by

reading about things in a history textbook,
but it happens to them every night in their
living rooms, the war in Vietnam, riots in
Europe?

Margaret Mead: They happen here and now, but, of course,
the immediacy is very much distorted by
the fact that the kids do not know which is
real and which is fictional. When Oswald
was shot, the adults were very upset; the
children were not initially upset, they
had to learn this reaction from the adults
because they do not know which is a
detective story and which is actuality.

Question: What about the adolescents, the college
kids, would they know the difference?

Margaret Mead: They learn quite early and they have learned
how to recognize the ads and they are very
sophisticated about it, but the small
children see a great deal of fictitious behavior on television as well as real things
and they cannot always differentiate.

Question: Would you say that another aspect of the
shared experience is that the youth may be
showing a trend or a model towards a common language?

Margaret Mead: Youths' common language is music and
they do not have to talk much. They can go
from country to country and smoke pot and
play and feel. Music is, of course, the easiest
common language to work with, but it is the
hardest to put into any form. To people who

have always depended upon words these youths appear anti-rational. People think that they are irrational, but really they are just anti-academic and in many ways anti-words.

Question: Another quote from your book *Growing Up in Samoa,* which also seems to me to be pertinent to contemporary youth problems, is the following: "For a new departure in the field of personal relations is always accompanied by the failure of those who are not strong enough to face an unpatterned situation. Canons of honour, of personal obligation, of the limits of responsibilities, grow up only slowly. And, of first experimenters, many perish in uncharted seas" (Mead 1928). Now this makes me think of the so-called hippies, the social dropouts, and some of these in fact have not been able to make their way in the uncharted seas. But you wrote this in 1928, when there were no hippies. Well, what is it that is not changing in the middle of what seems nowadays to be perennial rapid change? What are the basic experiences of youth that do not change?

Margaret Mead: Well, sex is a recurrent problem in every society and one can decide to let young people experiment and they can experiment covertly as long as they keep the doors shut, which was the situation in the 1920's, or one can chaperone them, which is a dreadful lot of work, or one can marry them off, by virtually child marriage, which is what we tried in the 1950's. We got everybody married that we could and the girls responded by getting pregnant as early as possible. What we did in the 1940's was to stop chaperoning; the young people had motor cars and chaperoning with motor cars was almost impossible, so that was the real reason why we gave it up. There was no way of stopping sex experimentation, therefore we decided that marriage was the solution.

Question: Is this what you are advising?

Margaret Mead: No, this is what society did. Society as a whole adopted the attitude of the mother of the lower socioeconomic class. This is another development which is very important, that is, the rise of lower-class standards as the principal standards of the whole society. In lower-class families, one got married when one had to. People experimented; in the 1950's, if a girl got pregnant she got married, and thus we had this mass of married college students, partly patterned on the GIs who were married. The students lived in trailers and had babies. This resulted in a new kind of style which was followed through the 1950's. Colleges would say, "Well the only reason we have dormitories is because we do not have enough married students' quarters," and so the adult world said, "Very well, we still disapprove of sex, we still think that it should be within marriage and, if you get pregnant, then we will let you get married." Then we had a few colleges left who still used to throw students out if they were pregnant. But in most colleges, if Suzie said she was pregnant and would like to be married in the college chapel next week, everybody approved, so that we produced a degree of hypocrisy that was unbelievable. Now, the kids say, "We are just sick of this," and the population explosion idea came, and they got the pill, and they said, "O.K. now we can tell you that we will not have children and we are going to live together, and we are not going to get married until we feel the marriage is good." Adults still believe that marriage can be final which, of course, is nonsense. The young people are saying to adults, "Please provide us with nice upholstered furniture for us to make love on, we are tired of the back seats of cars," and they are making the colleges provide the coeducational dormitories where boys can stay in girls rooms and girls can stay in boys rooms. And they wrested this freedom from the adult world.

Question: How did this generation succeed in wresting things that ours could not?

Margaret Mead: Well, it never occurred to us to want it for one thing. Our notion was that one got the adult world to stay out of one's hair, but one did not expect adults to underwrite one's experimentation. Members of this generation have experienced affluence. They say we do not want to go to college anyway;

they say, "If you insist that we go, we're young adults, we have a right to sex experience." Two generations have been influenced by Freud and others, who kept telling people that sex was necessary. Now, in the United States, we think that sex is like digestion—and constipation is bad for you—and if people did not have some sex all the time, something would go wrong. So the adults feel more and more guilty in denying sex to the young people from whom they are demanding longer and longer years of education. It is really a breakdown in the style of adult morality.

Question: On the subject of drugs, do you see the use of drugs by young people as a manifestation of the dependence of adults on all drugs including alcohol?

Margaret Mead: The young think that they have a better drug—they prefer pot to alcohol. Pot makes one peaceful instead of making one fight; it creates group feeling and at the same time a certain type of distance. People have had to get drunk to stand the nightmares of social events experienced by business groups in which wives had to accompany their husbands. Today the young believe that one can just smoke a little pot and turn on some music and get through the evening (one does not even have to play bridge).

Question: It has been said that pot is a far more

civilized drug than alcohol, would you agree with this?

Margaret Mead: Yes, I certainly would agree with it, but we have set it up, we have made a trap for ourselves because we have called pot a narcotic and so we have made it related to heroin and LSD and everything else. We have made it the road to heroin. Chemically it is not, but we have made it so socially.

Question: Because it's illegal and one has to go underground?

Margaret Mead: Underground, and because the young were told that it was addictive. When they discovered that it was not addictive, they decided to try something else and something else.

Question: One complaint that is often made, and not just by young people but by people who are looking into the whole marijuana history, is that because young people have realized that a lot of what was said about marijuana was often false, and sometimes frankly dishonest, they say, "You did not tell us the truth about pot and therefore we will find out ourselves about the other drugs."

Margaret Mead: I believe a lot of that is true. The only people whom the young will listen to now are their age mates who have tried the other drugs. I think that the only way out of this drug dilemma now is to let the young people pull themselves out.

Question: Of course when somebody like yourself says in public, "Let us legalize the substance and let kids over 16 take it," people are stunned and say, "There must be something with Margaret Mead, maybe she is getting old," how do you react to this?

Margaret Mead: People are certainly going to say that I am getting old when they do not like what I say. I have been saying the same things for years. It is interesting how they react, but it is also interesting *when* they react.

I get maybe two hundred letters on a controversial point, about a hundred very pro and a hundred very anti and nothing in between, because people apparently only write letters when they are having fits. When I first looked at two or three of the negative letters, I thought, "Why do people have to be so hostile," but when I looked at the pro letters I found them just as ridiculous. One person says, "You should be executed like the Rosenbergs," and another person says, "I can't imagine a world without Margaret Mead." These are equally crazy.

Question: It has been said that the drug issue, and particularly the marijuana issue, has come to symbolize the concerns and worries of the adults and the impatience and despair of the youth. Do you think this is true?

Margaret Mead: In the past there have been battles between adults and youth over every kind of indulgence. There was one over drinking, which everybody has now forgotten. In the United States in the 1950's an enormous amount of youths drank. The adults used to say, "You are too young to drink, just wait, and when you are 21 you can do as you like." But with marijuana the adults said that the young could never have it. On their side, they were locking youth out just as much as youth were locking them out. This symbolized the real break and it was different from the little boys smoking the corn-silk cigarettes behind the barn.

Question: At what age do you think marijuana should be made legally available, would you say over 16?

Margaret Mead: Well actually I did not suggest over 16. What happened was that somebody asked, "At what age do you think it would be safe to use it?" and I replied, "If for alcohol the age limit is 18, I think that pot is about two years less harmful." But I think if we repealed the laws against marijuana, we would control it the way we control tobacco and alcohol and about as successfully. The real danger is that if we allow the present situation to continue people will get used to handling marijuana illegally.

Question: Are we in fact controlling it now?

Margaret Mead: No, we are not controlling it at all, we are just frightening and penalizing people; we are using the control against anybody —the children of political figures; we are using it as straight blackmail, everywhere, all the time.

Question: The present drug sitaution appears to have a lot of similarities to the Prohibition Era in the United States—there is underground traffic, organized crime. . . .

Margaret Mead: And the racketeers and the corruption of politicians. We have never recovered from Prohibition and now things are worse and the only way that we could correct them is by making necessary changes in the present law. It is most unlikely that this will happen in the near future. The kids who have taken drugs and do not like them, and there are enough of them now, could convince other kids; this also could help the situation. We are beginning to pass laws to permit any youngster over 12 to go to a clinic without the parents' permission.

Question: Do you think this reflects a change of attitude of adults towards the young?

Margaret Mead: But you see what we are doing, we will have to change all those laws which we passed to protect juveniles. We will have to get rid of the old-style Juvenile Court; we will have to knock out the juvenile detention home. All the laws that were originally passed to protect kids do not protect them anymore. And this is very hard on the adults; everything the adults planned 50 years ago has boomeranged.

Question: Can you give us some examples of this?

Margaret Mead: Yes, Juvenile Courts now are moving to give juveniles defense lawyers, but the objective of the Juvenile Court was to take the juveniles out of the adversary system, to have no public hearings and no criminal record. Now we are demanding defense lawyers in Juvenile Court because the children have to be protected against the way that the society is treating them. For example, a high-school principal tells a boy that he cannot come to school if he does not cut his hair, therefore in order for him to be able to grow his hair as he likes, there has to be a legal decision, that he has rights, and so now school children are being given legal rights. Even unborn babies are being given legal rights. In Washington, D.C., a mother, who was a member of some religious sect, refused blood transfusions. The doctor said that she and the baby would die without the transfusion, but she refused to have it and the Court declared that she must have it for the baby's sake and the mother was given a compulsory blood transfusion. Now this is turning everything upside down. We also have in the United States, and in most industrialized countries, the revolt of all the people who are "being done good to"—the people on welfare, students, parishioners, prisoners, mental patients, unmarried mothers.

Question: What on the whole do you think the reaction of members of the caretaker professions would be in the face of this rebellion?

Margaret Mead: They are angry and they are aggrieved. Professionals dedicate their lives. With the exception of a few physicians at the end of long training, none of them makes much money. A sign of being good, of course, in our society is for a professional not to make much money.

Question: Do you think that it would be necessary for the professionals to restructure their professional identities, their roles, their places in the hierarchy, their privileges, their prerogatives? This is all being challenged now.

Margaret Mead: It's asking a terrible lot and it is worse in hospitals, where the authority position has been based on the responsibility for life and death. At the center of the medical hierarchy was the responsibility of the doctor and when the neighborhood comes in and takes over a hospital or a clinic it is terrifying to the people who have been training young doctors all of their lives to take this responsibility.

Question: I can see for the general physician and surgeon this responsibility for life and death. What has been the responsibility of the psychiatrist?

Margaret Mead: Well, of course he always had trouble in this context because he never had clear-cut responsibilities except in suicide cases. When there is no suicide threat the patient gets a little better or no better under his treatment. He has to work in a social context and thus the social worker and the psychiatrist are vis-à-vis with the doctor and the nurse. The doctor and the nurse could afford the kind of arrogance that went with clearcut responsibility, but that does not apply in the case of the psychiatrist and the social worker.

Question: Some people have acknowledged the criticisms and the striking idealisms of the youth of the 60's, but they believe that the idealism is real and that when these young people become adults and take on the responsibilities of providing for others and of carrying out some service in society they will become just as conservative as previous generations. What do you think?

Margaret Mead: But the problem is not about being conservative. People keep looking at a few radicals among the youth and thinking that this is the point. In the United States 4 percent of the college students are activists, but 60 to 70 percent of the students agree on the goals; they simply disagree on the means. I grant that people change as they grow older and have more responsibilities, but these youths will never see the world the way the adults did. It is the way of looking at the world that has changed; it is the difference between thinking one can win wars and knowing that one cannot. We have radicals and conservatives, the responsibles and the irresponsibles. The ones who pick the helping professions, who pick teaching, or who pick medicine, are going to be, of course, the more responsible people and the more concerned, but none are going to undergo a change back to the old adult way of looking at things.

Question: You say that a large percentage of the students, say around 60 percent, agree with the aims and the philosophy of the radicals. Does this in part explain why, during relatively tranquil times on campuses, it is only a small group who acts, but when the law-enforcement agencies come in, as we saw at Columbia and following the shooting recently at Kent State, it is as if suddenly the majority of the student body become activists?

Margaret Mead: They all become activists, not because they are interested in the bombs and these things, but because they are on the other side.

Question: So in a way they are allowing the small minority to act?

Margaret Mead: Revolutions are always made by minorities, but if they do not have a large group backing them for whom they are speaking and if the other side has not lost faith there are no revolutionary results. Now what has happened on our campuses is that the faculty lacked sufficient faith in the system to stand up against the onslaught and did not know how to handle it. There were strikes and violent confrontations. In the spring of 1970, although there was a strike there was no trouble at Columbia. This is because the students were not there, they were out in the communities working and listening and talking to the construction workers and to Congressmen in Washington and to all kinds of people. There were few on the campus. There were two or three little episodes; somebody put a bomb under Alma Mater but this was an individual act—the person who did it was probably disturbed or psychotic. We should get things set up so that the acts of psychotic individuals or very small groups of disturbed people do not trigger large disturbances.

Question: What type of controls or prophylactic techniques were you thinking of to prevent the act of a single disturbed individual from escalating into a mass disturbance?

Margaret Mead: For one thing the public has got to learn to discriminate between a single act of arson by a disturbed person and a plan by a student group. We have also got to stop escalating the climate of opinion. This is what television and other media have to learn. They have to become more responsible; they have to stop giving such a disproportionate amount of time to violence and if they do not we will continue to have this atmosphere.

Question: You have said that you do not think that these young people will change their view of the world when they grow older. What will they be like as parents? Would you like to speculate as to what approaches they will use to child rearing that might be different from the way they themselves were brought up?

Margaret Mead: I think they will get rid of the divine right of parents. For example, if a mother told her child to sit still and if he asked why, the answer would be: "Because I told you to, you do as I tell you because I am your mother." I expect that the young as parents will explain to their children why they are told to do certain things, which is the way I brought up my own child.

Question: Do you feel that there has been a tendency in the last decade for parents and families to delegate or abandon a lot of their traditional responsibilities and roles to institutions in society?

Margaret Mead: We do delegate a good deal of responsibility to the school, especially in the United States where there were millions and millions of European peasants. These parents were incapable of giving their children proper direction; many of them were illiterate and unable to speak the language, but they wanted their children to speak English, to learn American styles of living and the schools did the greater part of this job. But the schools have their problems. If the schools try to teach anything with a heavy ethical element they get into trouble. We should never have had the row that we had about prayer in the schools, we should simply have had silent prayer. Parents could have told their children to repeat the alphabet if this is what they wanted. But the parents still have the notion that whatever it is, once it is taught in schools, it has to be in accordance with sanctified moralities, sanctioned by churches. I think my statment about marijuana caused such a stir because it was made to a Senate Committee. There are people in the United States who think that a Senate hearing is somehow part of the Establishment and sanctioned by God. The word *legalized* to a large number of our population means *sanctified*. They are the people who have been passing laws for 400 years to make other people do what they want them to do, thus you suggest legalizing something and they think it means that you sanctified it. For example, consider the fight about sex education in schools. The teacher tells the children that they can say a word they have never been allowed to say in school before and the parents are shocked—not because the children are going to get new information for those parents know just as well as anybody else that the kids are going to pick it up on the street. But to most parents, school remains a sanctified place, not a center for learning new ways.

Question: In North America our understanding of the psychologic and sociologic development of the adolescent and youth has been based primarily on psychodynamic schools, specifically psychoanalytic schools, which have taught and still teach that it is necessary and normal to have rebelliousness and turmoil as part of the normal adolescent growth pattern. Now recently some of the research with normal high-school kids has brought this very much in doubt. Would you go so far as to say that an adolescent who does not go through turmoil and rebelliousness is possibly abnormal?

Margaret Mead: Well it depends on the period, the society and the class. In the United States we gave up weaning adolescents. The adolescent went from a state of adolescent dependency in the home to marriage; he went from one family to another and never went through a process of young adulthood. The American family weans very early, to the degree that it will not stand an adolescent in the home, especially a girl; as soon as the girl shows any signs of puberty her mother wants her to get out and she is ejected. She marries the first boy who will marry her. One can call this turmoil. There is a critical period at the point where children reach puberty, and they are reaching it earlier than formerly—four months earlier per decade—so that puberty is hitting where once latency hit. In the time of the American Revolution, on the average, young adults were six years later reaching puberty than they are now.

Question: To what extent, do you feel, adult professionals working with youth find the youth-
ful rebelliousness and challenging of tradi-
tions and value useful in redefining their
own changing roles?

Margaret   Well one cannot redefine one's role if one
Mead: does not continuously listen to the young.
We did some studies several years ago,
in which we took groups of very intelligent,
highly educated adults in their 70's and 80's,
who were reading and attending literature
classes. We divided these into two groups,
those who were staying close to their grandchildren and those who were not. Through
observing the two groups we learned that
the only way one can recycle oneself is with
the help of the young. This becomes especially important in a rapidly changing
society such as ours.

Question: Is this something which tends to happen
spontaneously or something which requires
conscious effort?

Margaret   We know that it requires a conscious effort
Mead: because there are not any grandchildren
around automatically. To a degree it still
happened spontaneously, say in the early
part of the century, because people were
not so mobile and the grandparents were
around.

Question: Do you think that there are youth workers
and people who work with disturbed chil-

dren who have a dislike of parents and of the Establishment?

Margaret Mead: Yes, there are and it is changing now because we are beginning with a whole new generation. We have lots of young men from Ivy League colleges teaching small children. They may be doing this as a way of getting out of the draft, but I would not call that a neurotic need, they would rather serve society than to go to Vietnam.

Question: In the last five years it has become increasingly difficult to attract bright college graduates to business. What significance do you attach to that?

Margaret Mead: Business is also discovering that the young people they do attract have exactly the same ideas as the others. They are going into business with the notion that they are going to make business more responsible. The young are looking for points of leverage in the society and some of them see that business has tremendous leverage. They know that businesses are institutions like any other and that one can change them. They are joining with the idea of changing them.

Question: Why do you think the young today are more concerned about the quality of life rather than the material technologic process?

Margaret Mead: These are the children who have been smothered with things, whose parents did not have much when they were young and bought them thousands of plastic toys that broke. The child who had really beautiful toys, which were well made, does not turn out to be so materialistic. It is the anti-materialism of people to cheap materialism. These are the people who are turning against what they call materialism and want a simpler life.

Question: The blue-collar workers seem to think that these kids are pampered and spoiled and do not appreciate the advantages they have had. Do you think the blue-collar workers are a part of the so-called silent majority?

Margaret Mead: Certainly, the silent majority is the lower middle class; they are the backbone of any fascist movement. They have just arrived at where they are, but their financial situation is precarious. They are the ones who live in the suburbs; they are not the ones who live in a cold-water flat with twelve kids. It is the blue-collar worker who drives a Cadillac who resents the present youth. He is living way beyond his means. He does not know where he is going to get the money to pay the mortgage; he is threatened by inflation. He hates everybody who came to this country or who arrives after he did because he is afraid that they will invade his position and take it away from him. This is, within limits, true of the lower middle class everywhere.

Question: One is struck with the similarity in dress, fads, music, philosophy and so on among youth around the world. Is this just a simple matter of group identification because they see each other on television or does it go deeper than that?

Margaret   Well, I think they are all facing the same
Mead: problem, wherever they came from. Whether they came from the center of New Guinea or the center of London, it does not seem to matter that their parents and grandparents come from different backgrounds and cultures.

Question: You have pointed out that the concept of stages of development in civilization and thinking of some civilizations as primitive, others as more civilized, is no longer valid. Can you elaborate on this?

Margaret   We used to think that a society had to go
Mead: through a long series of stages, but this is not true any more. It used to take a very long time to make any changes at all, then change speeded up. Now we have a society which involves the whole planet. It does not make any difference where you come from, you end up with a transistor radio. In the past, when you came out of the stone age, you did not read the London Times, you went to a native school, you learned a little bit of language, and then members of the next generation learned a little bit more and maybe they went to a very inferior school.One could not become an intellectual

in one generation. Today everybody is sharing all kinds of knowledge and experience.

Question: It has been said that there has been a true or relative permissiveness in the upbringing of the current youth generation. Experts have been blamed for preaching this permissiveness, but what made the parents bring up the children according to manuals?

Margaret Mead: Well, because in our rapidly changing world, in an immigrant society, it was not only child rearing that had to be learned but also what kind of curtains to put up and what to wear and how to use the telephone. We have always in this society written manuals for adults on how to behave, because adults cannot be taught in the same way that children are taught. Respect for adults is shown by writing a manual about how to bring up children. The immigrants came to this country as adults, and because they had to learn new styles they got used to learning nearly everything from a book.

Question: As a result of people saying that there has been too much permissiveness it has been suggested that we have got to stop it. Now to me it seems rather absurd to think that with a group of kids who may have been brought up in a laissez-faire manner we could suddenly change direction. Should we wait till the next generation?

Margaret Mead: No, we cannot wait for the next generation, we do not have any time to wait for the next generation.

Question: What is a generation these days, how many years?

Margaret Mead: They run around 10 now and, after all, the age of puberty for girls is down to 10 and it is this falling age of puberty that is part of the changing generation gap. No, we cannot wait and the best way to change one generation is to change the methods of bringing up the next. It is not a question that the babies are going to be different, but that the mothers are going to be different.

Question: What advice should we professionals give to the parents?

Margaret Mead: Parents have to get some understanding of looking at a baby as a growing human creature who is living in a world that they did not live in—he is in a room with a television set. This is a different baby from the kind of baby that they were, both as an individual and as a member of a group, and they are going to have to listen and to pay attention as the child develops. They have to find out what he is really learning, instead of what people think he is learning.

Question: What about the teachers?

Margaret Mead: Well teaching is similar. If teachers cannot learn from the students, then they cannot teach.

Question: Professionals working with problem youth?

Margaret Mead: Here again these professionals have to go out and listen, listen to the kids and listen to them talk, so that they can find out what they are talking about and not use a nice little formula which will explain everything.

Question: Politicians. How should they learn from this recent youth generation?

Margaret Mead: The same way—talk to them, bring them in. A very prominent man in the United States who played a great role in some of our youth conferences and who has written a great deal about youth has said that he had not spoken to an undergraduate for 20 years. There are people in children's agencies who talk as if they had not seen a child for 20 years. Memory did all right when things were changing slowly. People did remember what a baby was like, but not today. Today, we need continuing experience.

REFERENCES

Mead, M. (1928): *Coming of Age in Samoa.* Dell Publishing Co., Inc., New York, p. 175.

Mead, M. (1939): *Growing Up in New Guinea.* William Morrow & Co., Inc., New York.

Mead, M. (1970): *Culture and Commitment.* Natural History Press, Doubleday & Co., Inc., New York.

Chapter 2

DEVELOPMENTAL PSYCHOLOGY OF YOUTH

Daniel Offer and Judith Offer

INTRODUCTION

Adolescence has often been characterized as the "in-between stage," when the boy is not quite a man or the girl still has so many childish qualities. A conceptualization of adolescence as a transitional stage characterizes it as a unique period of disruption and change. This theoretical framework focuses our subsequent observations onto personality changes and defensive maneuvers of the adolescent. The continuities of individual patterns of development and the qualities demarcating a relative stability of functioning within adolescence have already been discredited by the initial characterization. It is our thesis that adolescence should be understood *as a stage in itself,* and comparisons can be meaningful when one adolescent population is contrasted with another. Each cycle in life will bring new challenges and opportunities, but the changes will be incorporated into the basic personality structure. Our working definition of adolescence is as the stage of life that starts with puberty and ends at the time when the individual's independence from his parents has attained a reasonable degree of psychologic congruence. The beginning phase is obviously easier to define, although there is some difference of opinion as to which of the pubertal changes should be utilized to mark the beginning of adolescence. The end of adolescence is much more difficult to describe. Each new dissertation on late adolescence suggests ways of defining "reasonable" independence or utilizes other criteria which are equally difficult to define for delineating an end to adolescence.

The span of years devoted to adolescent development will vary in different cultures, and with different definitions. The term "adolescence" no longer is equivalent to "pubescence." The former is seen as the psychologic developments which are related to the biologic growth which the latter term is utilized to depict. In the last 50 years within Western cultures, adolescence has become a progressively longer stage. The concept of reasonable independence has been translated into financial independence and/or marriage. If these behavioral criteria are accepted, a high-school student who upon graduation begins work in a factory and marries at 19 experiences a shorter period of parental dependence than the individual who continues his education, attending college and graduate school, and is supported by his parents until the age of 26, marrying at 28.

In order to limit the scope of this chapter we have decided to concentrate on the years from 12 through 21. We discuss the reactions of adolescents to pubertal changes. The necessity for the adolescent to habituate himself to his changing body and to his changing needs is the one common denominator of all discussions on adolesence. The adolescent will also be reacting to the attitudes of the parent generation and of the cultural biases.

In the United States, adolescents are conspicuously grouped by their presence in a school setting. Twelve- to 14-year-olds are in junior high school. Most 14- to 18-year-olds are in high school. The term "teenager" is often used to refer to the high-school-age adolescent. The 18- to 21-year-old either begins full-time work, marries, or enters a university or professional school. He has been described as the "young adult," the "late adolescent," or the "post-adolescent." Individual variances as well as the specification of developmental tasks, the accomplishment of which predicates an ideal and the measurement of which requires the ideal tool, reveal the use of age limits as only arbitrary devices. We use them as aids for communication.

Certain developmental theories of adolescence are to be found repeatedly in comprehensive collections of essays. One author chooses an Eriksonian frame of reference; another stresses Piaget's cognitive development, while a third describes adolescence in terms of "object-loss" and "object-seeking" maneuvers. The language is different, thus obscuring certain of the differences between the various systematizations. Furthermore, the data available from empirical studies seem to be far too limited to be able to list, for example, four developmental tasks. There are too many populations as yet unsampled for us to be able to make generalizations about the whole. We shall evaluate what is written now, summarize data on one group of adolescents, and examine the issue which such evaluations have shown to be central to the clinician's understanding of the developmental psychology of adolescence. We discuss certain aspects of developmental psychology while emphasizing the importance of considering the theoretical positions as tentative and population-specific.

The conceptualization of the normative developmental psychology of adolescents has, to a large extent, depended upon the clinical experiences of psychiatrists and psychoanalysts with disturbed adolescents or juvenile delinquents. Thus, in the process of extrapolating from psychopathology to normative theory, it has been difficult for psychiatrists to focus upon the adaptive in human behavior. Despite the above, psychiatrists do engage in discussions about typical, average, or normal patterns of development. Their data, however, have been minimal.

The Normal Adolescent Project

In order to avoid such obvious methodological pitfalls, we began, in 1962, a longitudinal follow-up study on a group of nonpatient adolescents in two Chicago suburbs (see Offer, 1969). We intentionally selected a group of teenagers whose adaptation to their environment was not seen as deviant by parents, teachers, or our initial selection instruments. Subjects were selected on the basis of the *normality-as-average* perspective. (See Offer and Sabshin, 1966, for a detailed theoretical discussion of concepts of normality and mental health.) A typical or normal student was defined as one whose answers on our self-image questionnaire fell within one standard deviation from the mean in nine out of ten scales which described various aspects of adolescent functioning. The questionnaires were given to 326 entering freshmen boys in the two suburban high schools.

Two psychiatrists, Drs. Offer and Marcus, have been interviewing the 73 males selected. The project is in its eighth year. The subjects are now 4 years post-high school. In addition to the psychiatric interviews of the adolescents, the subjects were given psychologic testing twice (at the ages of 16 and 20). Parents were also interviewed. Teachers completed rating scales on the adjustment of the students. The same interdisciplinary team of researchers studied the development of 30 female adolescents (Offer and Offer, 1968).

In this chapter we will utilize our data on the developmental psychology of our normal subjects as an example of how one group of adolescents passes through adolescence. It should not be construed to mean that we are unaware of the limitations of our data. There are many other samples of normal adolescents in other socio-, cultural, ethnic, and religious settings. However, we believe that generalizations about development are meaningless if the specifics from which the generalizations were made are not identifiable. Thus, our data will identify the reasons for our positions.

The chapter is divided into four sections: (1) Sexual Behavior; (2) The Adolescent and His Parents; (3) Adolescent Turmoil; and (4) Identity.

SEXUAL BEHAVIOR

Developmental Issue

After the physical changes of puberty have taken place, the individual is biologically a sexually mature adult. Biologic development and emotional readiness for heterosexual relationships do not proceed at the same pace. Though the sexual impulses are present with increasing strength, there exist psychosocial blocks which do not allow for discharge of these urges. What happens to the sexual impulses and when is the "correct" time for their expression are questions which have plagued many investigators and theoreticians in the field of adolescent psychiatry and psychology.

Relevant Data

The high-school students participating in our research project were free to discuss sexual feelings during any of the interviews. However, the male adolescents rarely spoke about sexual incidents when asked in one of their sophomore-year interviews when they had experienced feelings of shame, guilt, depression, and anxiety. The sixth interview, which occurred during the teenager's junior year at high school, was devoted to questions about heterosexual relationships. The adolescent males might blush and then answer our questions, adding questions of their own. In discussing heterosexual behavior more than in any other area of discussion, these teenage subjects would ask what others had told us.

The cardinal findings are that there was a discrepancy of several years between the time our adolescent subject was biologically able to produce children and the time the adolescent engaged in intensive heterosexual activities. In this sense, the male adolescent subject was "slow" in becoming involved sexually with a female. Ten percent of our study population had sexual intercourse by the end of high school. The rate rises to 30 percent by the end of the first post-high-school year, and 50 percent by the end of the third post-high-school year.

Although the teenager was uncomfortable when he talked about his own sexual feelings and impulses, he liked to appear "liberal" when talking about such issues as premarital sex. The high-school student generally thought that sexual intercourse was "okay" after high school. Interviewer: "Why not sooner?" Student: "The girl might become pregnant." Interviewer: "There are contraceptive methods available." Student, flushing: "Well, we're just not mature enough to handle 'it' yet, and teenagers *should* wait until they are old enough."

The adolescent male in early and mid-adolescence was not as worried about his participation, or lack of it, in heterosexual activities as were our female subjects in the concomitant study which we undertook. For the male, learning to curb his aggressive impulses is more important than learning to handle his sexual impulses. When he acts out, it is most often aggressively, in delinquent or violent behavior. In contrast, the adolescent female is more preoccupied with sex and the girl who does act out is likely to utilize the sexual route.

Many questions during our interviews would elicit blushing or seductive behavior, but the female adolescent, particularly, wanted to talk about her sexual attitudes and fears. Her fantasy life is vivid, and kissing a boy for the first time may be equivalent unconsciously to becoming pregnant. Gratification from fantasy life aids the female in handling her sexual impulses and in experimenting in thought with her changing and eroticized body without the massive guilt feelings which are as yet associated with heterosexual activities.

Dating was considered as part of the social format. The adolescent wanted to do the right thing. The female's concern with her place in the social field gave rise to questions like, "Am I popular?" or "Am I attractive?" much more than, for example, "What kind of feelings do I have towards a specific girl or boy?" Though the action is often limited, whatever does occur attains significance for the adolescent and her self-image. We asked a 15-year-old girl when she had experienced shame. Answer: "When I did something terrible with a boy." She had told only her best girl friend about what she had done and she would tell us no more. In another interview two years later, she revealed that the "terrible thing" had been kissing a boy. Apparently for this subject at age 17, to kiss a boy was no longer as great a sin as it was at 15.

Theoretical Implications

Have new cultural mores revolutionized today's sexual practices?

Recent empirical studies on adolescents and young adults do not support claims of increased sexual experiences for today's adolescents as compared to those of past generations. Our data on heterosexual behavior are consistent with our results from our questionnaire which has been given to 800 boys and 400 girls. Our results are also consistent with those of Reiss (1961), Douvan and Adelson (1966), and Simon, Lagnon and Carns (1968). For the teenagers studied, adolescent sexuality remained an emotional taboo as well as an environmental one. Even a complete revamping of sexual codes might not necessarily lead to earlier, less inhibited, and "healthier" sexual adjustments. It would take a more global shift in environmental and psychologic conditioning of these adolescents.

What does seem to be changing more than the practices is the openness of discussing sex. Interviews of adolescents conducted within the context of studies on non-patient populations indicate that adolescents welcome the opportunity to talk about sexual feelings and experiences. Could this be another way of handling the impulses which were formerly reported as a subject of conversation of peer groupings on street-corners?

The inexperienced adolescent must formulate new rationale to aid him in proceeding at his own pace toward heterosexuality. Since the advent of modern contraceptive methods, the adolescent who feared that intercourse would lead to pregnancy must develop other reasons for postponing sexual intercourse. In addition, prevalent cultural mores can exaggerate or ameliorate the adolescent's responses to his changing self. Newspaper and television reporting as well as classroom discussions and theoretical dissertations on the freedom of today's youth to engage in sexual activities may accentuate the abstaining teenager's belief that he (or she) is abnormal or, at least, inferior in comparison with his peers. His choice of defenses, be they adaptive or maladaptive, will be at least partially determined by cultural factors of his own and his parents' generations.

Perhaps as a reaction to the glorification of "free sex" as an answer to our neuroses, theoreticians of adolescent development have been underscoring the dangers of proceeding toward heterosexuality when biologic readiness is not matched by emotional readiness.

Deutsch tells us of a seminar in which Freud suggested the value of delayed sexual activities (Deutsch, 1967, p. 24): "Years ago, Freud, in a meeting that was limited to a small number of participants, expressed his opposition to Wilhelm Reich's insistence that sexual activity should begin in adolescence—that is, as soon as the biological readiness is manifested. Freud regarded the postponement of gratification as an important element in the process of sublimation and thereby essential to development."

Deutsch (1967) confirms the importance of the early same-sex relationships and warns of the disadvantages of early sexual gratification replacing too rapidly the homosexual friendships. In a discussion on female adolescents, she states: "I consider those girls who are involved prematurely in 'free love' as not the victors but the victims of the rebellious adolescent society. A great number of them are still involved in their earlier relationships with girlfriends. They 'fool around,' as the saying goes, with boys—but it is still with a side glance at the girls, and the heterosexual activity actually shows very little inner participation."

Deutsch later describes the case of Nora who could not decide which of three boys she preferred: "All three of the boys concerned were directly connected with her high school past; two of them were brothers of her old girlfriends; the third had had a mild affair with another of her friends from back home. This information was sufficient for me to understand that the homosexual attachments of her earlier adolescence had not yet been fully resolved and had in fact continued into her present pseudoheterosexual relationships."

Blos (1962) describes a type of frantic heterosexual activity which is defensive. For the female, he explains this in terms of the preoedipal attachment to the mother which is now revived. "The pseudoheterosexuality of this type of delinquent girl serves as a defense against the regressive pull to the preoedipal mother, that is, against homosexuality."

Erikson, (1968A) believes that sexual experimentation will provide a necessary part of identity-formation, but sexual pleasure need be preceded by a sense of one's own identity. The individual lacking a clear sense of who he is will be threatened by intimate relationships. In early and mid-adolescence, the teenager can concentrate his energies on less dangerous terrains, such as the football field or the classroom exam. There his emotional investments can be less intense and his disappointments more easily reversed.

THE ADOLESCENT AND HIS PARENTS

Developmental Issue

During adolescence, the individual must separate from his parent emotionally and intellectually. He must begin to know his own limitations and to utilize this knowledge in caring for himself. Ideally, the dependency characteristic of childhood should be relinquished. During adolescence, the former parent-child relationship shoud be changed sufficiently to allow the adolescent to proceed into a generational dyad in which he will be the primarily independent figure.

Profile of Jim: A Normal Middle-Class Suburban American Adolescent

At 11 years of age, Jim became increasingly argumentative. He disliked taking the garbage out every evening.

The problem for him was that he would feel guilty when he promised his mother he would empty the garbage and then would neglect to do it or would argue with his mother about why the job had to be his. He would also argue with his two brothers about which television program to watch or whose turn it was to do the dishes.

Jim would feel ashamed when his mother had to do things for him—like the times when he had a bad knee and Mother drove him to school, even though Dad disapproved of her chauffeuring.

Jim was an average student, considering a future in engineering. He was on his school's basketball team and very involved with the team members, the coach, practice sessions, and the big games. He began dating toward the end of his junior year in high school. His first date was for a party after the last basketball game of the season.

After high school, Jim went to a college 200 miles from his home. He thought all students should leave home after high school in order to learn to be on their own. During his freshman year, he was lonesome; he missed his mother's cooking and weekends with the family. He added: "It's not my parents that I need, but a girlfriend."

During summer vacations, he returned home. He had his hair cut a little shorter than was fashionable at his school in order to be able to secure a good summer job, working for a friend of his father's. He now enjoyed talking with his father more than previously. His father would invite Jim to join him for a drink. In general, Jim believed that both his parents treated him more like an adult since he had entered college. It did bother him when his mother would question him about his activities. He tended to reply in monosyllables (or less) and "get away" as soon as possible if she became "too prying."

Two years post-high school, he brought his girlfriend home to meet his parents and once brought her along to wait outside while the psychiatrist interviewed him.

During his junior year in college, he had sexual intercourse with a girl who was known to be "easy." He never dated her again, and felt that he had taken advantage of her.

At present, Jim is planning to go to graduate school in engineering or go into the army. He wants to spend next summer traveling.

Discussion of Data

As illustrated by Jim's behavior and the affect illicited within the interviews, Jim wanted to be accepted by his parents and admitted into their way of life but he wanted to do this with a feeling that he was acting as his own free agent. Jim was separating from his parents but without alienating them. During both Jim's high-school and college years, his parents expressed a pride in their son and his activities. The letting-go period was a gradual one. Conflicts were present but did not spiral out of control.

For the majority of students whom we studied, independence could be achieved without a total devaluation of parents. The adolescents studied in our normal population rarely rejected important parental values. Similarily, studies of student protesters and civil rights workers (Solomon and Fishman, 1964, Haan et al., 1968) have shown a congruence of parent-adolescent values.

The struggle for emotional disengagement was enacted in areas which could be seen as trivial to the adult eye. When the parent could keep the issue in perspective, the adolescent could achieve the victory needed for his sense of self-esteem. These "battles" could be won without a risk for the adolescent of having to jeopardize parental support. Even the issues chosen for the arguments were dependent upon parental preferences, but in a negative way. This has been conceptualized by Baittle and Offer (1970):

> When the adolescent rebels, he often expresses his intentions in a manner resembling negation. He defines what he does in terms of what his parents do not want him to do.

If his parents want him to turn off the radio and study, this is the precise time he keeps the radio on and claims he cannot study. If they want him to buy new clothes, the old ones are good enough. In periods like this, it becomes obvious that the adolescents' decisions are in reality based on the negative of the parents' wishes, rather than on their own positive desires. What they do, and the judgments they make, are, in fact, dependent on the parents' opinions and suggestions, but in a negative way. This may be termed a stage of "negative dependence." Thus, while the oppositional behavior and protest against the parents are indeed a manifestation of rebellion and in the service of emancipation from the parents, at the same time it reveals that the passive dependent longings are still in force. The adolescent is in conflict over desires to emancipate, and the rebellious behavior is a compromise formation which supports his efforts to give up the parental object and, at the same time, gratifies his dependent longings on them.

Our data also document the gradual shifts away from reliance on the parents. When the sport activities of high school terminate and the intensive home life of the younger adolescent dissipates, the adolescent must find substitute satisfactions. In follow-up interviews, the father of the male adolescent was mentioned much more frequently than had been true during early and mid-adolescence. Fewer,too, are the incidents of boys telling us that their mothers are beautiful or the unconscious shifting of the conversation to discussions about mother directly after the males were asked questions about their female peers. For certain males, the next stage was the period of taking out a girl in order to test the reactions of his parents. Finally, several of our subjects seem to be telling us for the first time of specific characteristics of their girlfriends.

The subjects are also relating to us the opinions and reactions of their peers more frequently in the post-high-school interviews. One male at age 16 told us that he agreed with his parents on the subject of the war in Viet Nam: "The Communists must be stopped or they will take over everything." Three years later he was at the conservative college of his choice. His political sentiments were unchanged except that replacing the comparison with the parental point-of-view was: "And I'm the most liberal guy on my campus." Meanwhile a more liberal former classmate at the radical college of his choice was berating himself for not having the "guts" to act on his principles and burn his draft card as certain of his more radical peers had done.

By the content of the subjects' responses, we could see the changes in interpersonal relationships. The adolescents were seeking out nonfamily members with whom they could share emotional experiences. There were some adolescents whose dependence upon parental figures had not altered significantly. For those adolescents whose development was delayed, the theoretical demarcation of an end to adolescence will be additionally complicated. Perhaps it will be marked by a rigidity of the earlier adolescent patterns, never transcended.

Implications for Theory

A. Freud (1958) writes: "There are few situations in life which are more difficult to cope with than an adolescent son or daughter during the attempt to liberate themselves."

Without erring in underestimating the conflicts which exist during adolescence, it is of importance to refrain from expecting momentous battles to characterize parent-adolescent relationships. In our study, parents and adolescents reported "bickering" during the early adolescent years. For the vast majority of our subjects, later difficulties failed to produce sustained feelings of misery or doom in either parent or adolescent.

The conflicts which do exist may be further encouraged by our own theoretical conceptualizations of relationships between the generations. Anthony writes (1969):

The adult in our Western culture has apparently learned to expect a state of acute disequilibrium and anticipates the "storm and stress" in his adolescent child as he once anticipated the negativism of his two-year old. The expectation has seemingly been incorporated into the literature of psychological development, and it may take methodical research and many years of endeavor to remove it from the textbooks. There is, however, growing support for the concept that society gets the type of adolescent it expects and deserves, and this is true of even those members who come into daily contact with the ordinary teenager.

This quote is found under a section labeled "The Stereotypic Response to the Adolescent as a Maladjusted Individual." One of A. Freud's (1969) recent articles is entitled: "Adolescence as a Developmental Disturbance."

In addition to the observation Anthony has made, it seems to us that the stereotype also has another effect. We have seen the parent (as well as the psychiatrist) who, expecting difficulties with adolescents, will minimize the importance of the problems which do exist, labeling them "normal" for the development of all adolescents. From parents who were interviewed while their sons were in high school, we heard frequent variations of the following sentiment: "We have some problems but our son is far better than most boys his age." The same parents had reacted more strongly to the negativism of their son when he was 11 and 12 years old. During their offspring's early adolescence, parents believed that precedents must be established for handling future conflicts, and they worried about what the future would bring if they were "already" having disagreements with their youngster. This outlook may contribute to the reporting by our subjects and their parents of greater disagreements during early adolescence than in the ensuing years. To a certain extent, rebellion has been sanctioned, institutionalized and encouraged for the later adolescent years. The interplay between cultural expectations and behavioral patterns constantly complicates the formation of neat stage-specific psychologic generalizations concerning behavioral patterns.

Are parental-adolescent conflicts inevitable? The adolescent must disengage himself from parental domination. He can do this without total renunciation of parental values, but rather through conflicts on minor issues which have been endowed with major importance for the adolescent's own growth and development. Battling between the generations need not characterize adolescence, as apart from other life stages when developmental tasks require infant, child, or adult to assert his independence from parental pressures. Adolescence, though, should be characterized by a significant emotional disengagement of the adolescent from the parent and a development of emotional relationships with others outside of the nuclear family complex. The emotional transfer to nonfamily members will, of course, never be complete; most importantly, the transfer of emotions must be accompanied by an emotional growth toward independence. Successful adaptation requires that the original preoedipal and oedipal conflicts be resolved sufficiently so that adult interpersonal relationships will not be a repeat of the former child-parent or adolescent-parent psychologic patterns. As the biologic and cultural situation changes, so should the psychologic variables retain their transactional role in the complex. If psychologic stagnation occurs, the effects will be manifested throughout the entire system.

ADOLESCENT TURMOIL

Intrapsychic Development: Review of Relevant Psychoanalytic Theory

Psychoanalytic literature describes adolescence as a time of psychologic imbalance when the functioning of ego and superego are severely strained. Instinctual impulses disrupt the homeostatic arrangements achieved during latency and inner turmoil results. Unresolved preoedipal and oedipal conflicts are revived; the repression characteristic of latency will no longer be sufficient to restore a psychologic equilibrium. The adolescent's intensive aggressive and erotic strivings are focused primarily upon parents and parent-figures. The physical, muscular, and hormonal growth of the adolescent endows the rearoused drives with a potency denied to the former child and frightening to the developing adolescent.

According to psychoanalytic theory, the strength of these aggressive and sexual impulses revived during adolescence necessitates an emotional disengagement from the nuclear family. However, the adolescent's value systems and self-esteem have been structured by internalizations of parental attitudes and behavior or, according to Grinker (1953), by the experiences of the infant in reaction to an influx of stimuli emanating from parents or parent-substitutes. To devaluate parents is to discredit also one's own internalizations gained from interactions with the parents. The adolescent's inner controls are loosened and his self-esteem fluctuating as he challenges the "truths" of his childhood. The reevaluation occurs at the same time as the adolescent's judgment and coping abilities are being weakened by demands of increased instinctual impulses.

The adolescent who now needs the support of strong, loving parents can least afford to accept that support. The loss of the parents as the supportive pillars of the individual's development has been conceptualized as "object-loss." According to Blos (1962), the primary theme of adolescence is the object-loss and the subsequent object-seeking. The adolescent depleted by his necessary rejection of dependency upon his parents must strive for narcissistic gratifications from deceptive magnifications of his own powers and from temporary identifications with peers and parental figures outside of the home. These defensive maneuvers are first steps in replenishing his strength.

This brief psychoanalytic conceptualization of early and mid-adolescence has been presented because we believe that psychoanalytic theory still provides the most comprehensive theoretical framework which we have today. If we accept it, the question arises as to how the adolescent manages to function during a period of such inner turmoil? Will he be likely to display behavioral contradictions? Will his psychologic state match that of the "as if" patient described by Deutsch (see A. Freud, 1936)? Will we be able to distinguish the symptoms of adolescence from symptoms displayed by the adult who has been diagnosed as suffering from a psychiatric disorder?

Given circumstances creating disequilibrium, the tendency of the living organism is to mobilize its forces toward a restoration of its equilibrium. Defensive maneuvers will be instituted in the service of adaptation to disquieting elements in the internal and external environment. Our question now concerns the affects experienced by adolescents and the character of the coping devices utilized. Additionally, through an examination of the organism's observable behavior, we can also gain information about the developmental requirements to which, it is postulated, the organism is reacting. Theory must be susceptible to revision from empirical examinations of the populations that the theory attempts to describe. Although our data from our Normal Adolescent Project may lack the depth of psychoanalytic patient data, it has the attribute of being collected from one segment of the nonpatient population whose psychologic development the above theory is designed to describe.

Relevant Data

To cope is to seek and utilize information under a variety of conditions in order to regulate behavior. Adolescence offers the individual an opportunity to test his defensive structure and/or his ability to cope. Our normal adolescent sample usually managed to cope with even severe stresses through their particular individual defensive structures and their action-orientation. When an unusual situation occurred, such as the death of a father, the adolescent would first deny the full emotional impact of the event. Then, he would cope with the stressful situation as well as the affect aroused by it through doing something. He would involve himself in time-consuming activities; often these activities were ones that would be necessitated by practical realities. Only slowly would he let himself experience the loss and mourn.

The stresses produced by the changes in body, in body image, and in emotional states were managed by these adolescents with little evidence of total personality upheavals or ascetic renunications of all bodily desires. As stated earlier, the male adolescent experienced the most difficulty with controlling his impulses during early adolescence. In mid-adolescence the involvement in sports, in cars, in hobbies, or on debating teams channeled his energies quite effectively. The girls, for whom culturally provided aggressive outlets were more limitetd, tended to handle these stresses in a more passive way by employing introspection or turning to close girlfriends with whom they could gain emotional satisfactions from hours of intimate discussions. For both sexes during late adolescence, there was a decrease in these types of sublimatory activities and an increase in heterosexual experiences.

Our normal subjects' action-orientation was coupled with a good sense of reality and a realistic self-image.

Their overall pattern of behavior was goal-directed, toward a future which they could envision and for which they were making mental time-schedules. Although they had questions concerning their vocational choices, most of these adolescents have been following their plans with surprisingly few obstacles.

Psychologic patterns of coping have retained an underlying similarity as different problems to be mastered have emerged. We see variations on a theme rather than extreme shifts in behavioral patterns. At 11 years old, George was fighting for his rights in reaction to a Boy Scout master's false accusation that he had started a fight; at 20 years old, George was being accused of taking drugs even though, he reports, he was an innocent by-stander, in no way involved in any illegal activities. His interest in painting, the family avocation, had remained constant, and he retained a good grade average. He associated with many of his peers but never had any particularly close friends.

Implications for Theory

Research on this group of normal adolescents does not validate psychologic conceptualizations of extreme turmoil characterizing adolescent development (see also Masterson, 1967, for similar findings). We base this judgment upon observations of patterns of behavior of adolescents and the meaning of these patterns to the individuals participating in our Project. The nature of turmoil is not such as to be able to keep itself hidden from the world, while presenting a picture of flexibility and good control over reality. In the segment of the adolescent population which we studied, behavior which might be considered as radically deviant by general American middle-class cultural standards was the exception rather than the rule. In home and school, the majority of these adolescents displayed an over-all pattern of consistency. Our follow-up studies on the adolescents have revealed a continuity of individual personality structures throughout the stages of adolescence (Offer, Marcus and Offer, 1970).

This being the case, we challenge the concept of great inner turmoil, swift mood swings, or other seemingly pathologic symptomatology as being a *necessary* part of adolescence. The turmoil experienced by our subjects is quantitatively different from the turmoil experienced by patient and delinquent populations seen in our hospital clinics and described in psychiatric case reports. The rebellion which we see in our research subjects and the emotional conflicts and crises that are both seen and postulated point toward theoretical conceptualizations of at least one type of normal adolescent with a lower level of turmoil than indicated in much of accepted psychiatric theory. We have studied our subjects for 8 years now, and have found no evidence to suggest that they are withdrawn, underdeveloped, or inhibited adolescents.

Interestingly, investigators who have spent most of their professional lives studying disturbed adolescents stress the importance of a period of turmoil for the developmental growth of the individual, while investigators who, like us, have studied normal adolescent populations find a minimal amount of turmoil displayed during the growth processes of many members of their research samples. We believe that the development of many adolescents can be better characterized by a concept of gradual shifts than by volcanic eruptions. Possibly, their clasp onto their parents was not so tight as to require a quick, total withdrawal for success in development.

Data on nonpatient populations suggest that adolescents can meet the requirements of emotional disengagement from internalized parental images and of pubertal growth spurts without displaying gross behavioral aberrations. In fact, the latter would, in adolescence as well as in other life stages, indicate a need for psychiatric evaluation and treatment. Neurotic symptomatology during adolescence should not be regarded as something the adolescent will "grow out of." According to Masterson (1967), diagnostic problems for the psychiatrist evaluating the adolescent relate to difficulties in classifying the sickness of the adolescent, not in determining its presence or its durability.

Once again, though, we must be sure to define adolescent behavior by norms for adolescents within similar cultural contexts and stages of biologic maturity. An explanation of the adolescent's behavior by comparisons with the child's or the adult's ignores the particular context of the tasks of adolescence and will result in more theories which regard the adolescent's normal behavior as being abnormal.

IDENTITY

Developmental Issue

The crystalization of identity is one of the developmental issues of adolescence. As conceptualized by Erikson (1968A) it is not one specific process but rather the culmination of many events which lead to: (1) a conscious sense of one's own individual identity; (2) an unconscious striving for a continuity of personal character; (3) a criterion for the silent doings of ego synthesis; (4) a maintenance of an inner solidarity with the groups' ideals. It has never been stated specifically when, in adolescence, identity conflicts either rise or should be resolved, though it has often been assumed that the answer to the question "Who am I?" has to come in late adolescence.

Relevant Data

Within our subject population, Jack is an example of a subject who had some identity conflicts. He revealed an array of contradictory plans and goals but the contradictions did not appear especially disturbing to him. At 20 years old, he thought he might become a history professor, a social worker, or an athletic coach. When the psychiatrist indicated that Jack's plans were not too concrete, Jack momentarily retreated: "Well, I might not even finish college." Immediately afterwards, though, he presented still other alternatives. He even suggested living a couple of years in Alaska after telling us that he had left the northern college which he had first attended because of his aversion to cold weather.

Andy on the other hand had planned his future long in advance. He was inclined toward introspection, depression, and a certain degree of rebelliousness. He retained consistent control over his life so that he was able to compensate for his disappointments through experiences which were highly satisfactory to him. An accurate self-appraisal allowed Andy to proceed according to his plans.

Our emphasis in our book, *The Psychological World of the Teen-Ager,* has been on the recognition of more than one route through adolescence. At present we can see three groups within our subject population. Subjects who, like Andy, tended toward introspection and depression are now adapting themselves to the demands of young adulthood. Others remain dependent upon their parents, or may be gradually shifting the dependency to male or female peers. For them, a sense of their identity may be delayed or never experienced. A third group belong to the category described by Erikson as young people in whom the identity crisis is a noiseless one (Erikson, 1968B). For those subjects the tasks of adolescence are being met without overt self-dissatisfaction or excessive narcissism. Of necessity, further definition of routes through adolescence must await further evidence of the development of our subjects.

The identity conflicts experienced by the vast majority

of our subjects range from mild to moderate. We have seen only a few subjects who manifested the Eriksonian type of identity crisis in which neurotic symptomatology becomes a temporary condition of normal development. The resiliency of the earlier self-confidence has continued for the majority of our subjects who feel satisfied with their choices and opportunities.

Implications for Theory

Our subjects can be understood in terms of Blos's (1967) concept of adolescence as the second stage of individuation, the first having been completed toward the end of the third year of life which was marked by rapid developmental progress toward the attainment of object constancy. Blos (1967) writes: "not until the termination of adolescence do self and object representation acquire stability and firm boundaries." Working within this framework which is, unfortunately, extremely difficult to measure empirically, we believe our subjects can be seen as approaching the end of the second stage of individuation. To what extent individuals ever completely separate from their internalized parental images and become firmly established in their own worlds of mature object representations is a variation of the question which we asked earlier when describing the difficulties of determining when adolescence terminates.

Late adolescence is portrayed as a time of delimitation in order to gain organization. The adolescent assumes adult responsibilities which are seen as limitations upon the scope of his activities and the freedom of his movement. However, the young adult who has successfully adapted to the biologic, psychologic and sociologic requirements of earlier stages of development will now be freer from the emotional conflicts which previously limited his world. Optimally, he is finding satisfactory ways of expressing himself, patterns for handling unresolved conflicts, which enable him to widen his horizons in ways that were impossible for him earlier when changing developmental tasks absorbed and restricted his energies to a greater degree. Thus, to conceive of adolescence as a stage of psychologic expansion to be terminated by the choices and limitations that proceed with the defining of oneself is not to present a complete picture. The process of defining oneself does not terminate with the termination of adolescence; what does happen is that the areas of focus and the meaningful interpersonal relationships of the future become manifest. If the passage through adolescence has been accomplished successfully, this focusing becomes as much a freedom to express oneself as it is a limitation to the mode for expression.

REFERENCES

Anthony, J. (1969): The reactions of adults to adolescents and their behavior. In: *Adolescence: Psychosocial Perspectives,* G. Caplan and S. Lebovici, Eds. Basic Books, Inc., New York.

Baittle, B. and Offer, D. (1970): On the nature of adolescent rebellion. In: *Annals of Adolescent Psychiatry.* S. Feinstein, P. Giovacchini, and A. Miller, Eds. Basic Books, Inc., New York.

Blos, P. (1962): *On Adolescence.* The Free Press of Glencoe, New York.

Blos, P. (1967): The second individuation process of adolescence. Psychoanal. Stud. Child 22:162–187.

Deutsch, H. (1967): *Selected Problems of Adolescence.* International Universities Press, New York.

Douvan, E. and Adelson, Y. (1966): *The Adolescent Experience.* John Wiley and Sons, Inc., New York.

Erikson, E. H. (1968A): *Identity: Youth and Crisis.* W. W. Norton & Co., New York.

Erikson, E. H. (1968B): Identity: Psychosocial. In: International Encyclop. of the Soc. Sc. 7:61–65. (Macmillan Co. and Free Press, New York.

Freud, A. (1936): *The Ego and the Mechanisms of Defemse.* International University Press, New York.

Freud, A. (1958): Adolescence. Psychoanal. Stud. Child 13:225–273.

Freud, A. (1969): Adolescence as a developmental disturbance. In:

Adolescence: Psychosocial Perspectives, G. Caplan and S. Lebovici, Eds. Basic Books, Inc., New York.

Freud, S. (1967): Quoted by H. Deutsch in: *Selected Problems of Adolescence*. International Universities Press, New York.

Grinker, R. R. (1953): *Psychosomatic Research*. W. W. Norton & Co., New York.

Grinker, R. R. (1962): Mentally healthy young males (homoclites). Arch. Gen. Psychiat. 6:405–453.

Haan, N., Smith, M. B. and Block, J. (1968): Moral reasoning of young adults: Political-social behavior, family background and personality correlates. J. Personality Soc. Psychol. 10:3, 183–201.

Masterson, J. F., Jr. (1967): *The Psychiatric Dilemma of Adolescence*. Little, Brown & Co., Boston.

Offer, D. (1969): *The Psychological World of the Teenager: A study of Normal Adolescent Boys*. Basic Books, Inc., New York.

Offer, D., Marcus, D. and Offer, J. L. (1970): A longitudinal study of normal adolescent boys. Amer J. Psychiat. 127:1.

Offer, D. and Offer, J. L. (1968): Profiles of normal adolescent girls. Arch. Gen. Psychiat. 19:513–522.

Offer, D. and Sabshin, M. (1966): *Normality: Theoretical and Clinical Concepts of Mental Health*. Basic Books, Inc., New York.

Reiss, I. L. (1961): Sexual codes in teenage culture. Ann. Amer Acad. Polit. Soc. Sci. 338:53–63.

Simon, W., Lagnon, J. and Carns, D. (1968): Sexual behavior of the college student. Paper read at the Academy of Psychoanalysis, New Orleans, Louisiana.

Solomon, F. and Fishman, J. R. (1964): Youth and race. J. Soc. Issues 20:54–73.

Chapter 3

PHYSICAL DEVELOPMENT: NEGLECTED DIMENSION

John R. Unwin.

> ...adolescents differ physiologically and psychologically from children and adults, and these differences should be better understood, more widely taught and more consistently remembered. Only when this has been done will it be possible to take adequate account of such factors as the rapid growth of adolescents, their high degree of activity, the interrelationship of their growth and their endocrine systems, and their requirements for a healthy personality development.
>
> World Health Organization 1965

There are so many areas in which professionals and others working with youth require at least a general knowledge of the phenomena involved in physical growth during this critical period of development; one thinks immediately of sex ("family life") education (Garell, 1968; Kirkendall and Calderwood, 1965; Schulz and Williams, 1969), unwed teenage mothers (Osofosky, 1968), assessment of variations in patterns of menstruation (Chiazze et al., 1968), venereal disease (King, 1966), acne, obesity, athletic performance and risks. It is thus striking to note that, despite such entreaties as those of the Expert Committee of the World Health Organization on Health Problems of Adolescence (World Health Organization, 1965), so few health and welfare (and educational) professionals seem to include physical status in their total evaluation of a given individual (Duche et al., 1966; Kestenberg, 1967; Unwin, 1970).

Yet youth (which I regard as stretching from the establishment of puberty until the attainment of a reasonable degree of economic and emotional independence by the early 20's) is a period during which the body, personality, intellect and social attitudes are developing erratically, usually independently of one another, and frequently explosively. The rate of physical growth during the spurt of the early teenage years is equaled only by that during the second year of life; previously unexperienced and intriguing abilities and sensations surface, sometimes with a speed and force which are disconcerting and even markedly threatening to the youth (and his family); and there is a wide variation in the age at onset, rate of change, and age at termination of the growth processes in the various body systems, such as bones, muscles, skin and sex organs.

Adequate descriptive material, including concise charts and tables, is available concerning the main phenomena involved, thanks to such researchers as Tanner (1962) in England; Gallagher (1966), Schonfeld (1969) and Reynolds and Wine (1948, 1951) in the United States; and various others (Lelong, 1957; Nellhaus, 1968; Stuart, 1946; Young, 1968). Duche and his co-authors (1966) point out that a reliable assessment of the stage of physical development of youth is "surprisingly easy, useful, but rarely done." This need not involve expensive equipment or highly specialized training—sufficiently accurate pubertal maturity ratings (Tanner, 1962; Young, 1968) can be attained from observation of the primary and secondary sexual characteristics, height, weight, and other signs, and unobtrusive techniques for evaluating physical maturity, while conducting routine physical and mental examinations, have been suggested (Levy, 1929; Schonfeld, 1969).

THE NORMAL SEQUENCE

As noted above, there is a wealth of practical descriptive literature giving all the information liable to be required by any professional or nonprofessional working with youth and wishing to evaluate biologic maturity (e.g., Reynolds and Wines, 1948, 1951; Schonfeld, 1969; Stuart, 1946; Tanner, 1962; Unwin, 1968). The present discussion will therefore limit itself to some broad observations which will help set the stage for a more detailed reading of the literature.

While the examination necessary to appreciate the stage of development of any individual youth requires only observation of relatively superficial parts of the body, it should be remembered that *all* growth phenomena (including in varying degree the intellect and personality) are dependent on, reflected in and closely monitored by internal hormonal and other physiologic processes (Donovan and Van der Werf Ten Bosch, 1965; Gardener, 1960; Johanson et al., 1969; Kestenberg, 1967; Weldon et al., 1967; Yen et al., 1969). And although the *sequence* of observable changes is the same for every normal youth, it must be stressed and taken into account in the assessment of individuals that there is a considerably wide range of normality for age of onset of puberty, and for the rate of change in the various body systems. It is in general better to err in the direction of generosity or "watchful expectancy" than to too readily label a slow maturer as abnormal.

During childhood and preadolescence, there has been a smooth rate of growth with little to indicate sudden change (apart from a slight mid-childhood spurt); there has been no underarm or pubic hair, the breasts have been flat and the penis and testes have not changed in size appreciably since infancy. Girls reach puberty some 2 years earlier than boys; hence initially the girls catch up with and then exceed the boys of the same chronologic age in respect to height and weight, the differences between the sexes for over-all size being most pronounced between the ages of approximately 11 and 13. Boys soon begin a phase of even more accelerated growth, however, and usually are taller and heavier than girls when fully mature. Both the intensity and the duration of the growth spurt are greater in males than in females. The abrupt growth spurt, suddenly changing the *rate* of ongoing growth, has a wide variation in its age of onset for different individuals, which explains why several youths of the same chronologic age can have a broad range of weight and height between them. The spurt in height, which occurs in mid-adolescence, precedes by several months the rapid increase in muscle size (which is, again, more pronouned in boys than in girls); once muscle growth commences, however, the strength of boys virtually doubles in about 4 years (Stuart, 1946).

As regards sexual changes, note that the onset of menstruation in girls follows the beginning of breast enlargement and the appearance of darkened pubic hair; the girl is sterile until some 1 to 3 years after the beginning of menstruation, because until then the monthly "periods" are not accompanied by the production of ova. In boys, the first ejaculation of semen follows the onset of accelerated growth of the penis by about 12 months, and the boy is not fertile until some 1 to 3 years after the first ejaculation— only then are enough mature sperm released to render impregnation of a female likely.

VALID ASSESSMENT OF STAGES
OF DEVELOPMENT

To speak of a 15-year-old or 18-year-old youth (that is, solely in terms of chronologic age) is virtually meaningless from any developmental point of view save that perhaps of intellect. The use of chronologic age as a standard for physical maturity is unreliable because of (1) the large variation in the age of *onset* of puberty and of the growth spurt; (2) the wide variation in the actual *rate* of growth from individual to individual during youth; and (3) the worldwide trend since the beginning of this century to-wards an earlier age of onset of puberty and the trend for youths to be increasingly taller and heavier than those of preceding generations (Canadian Family Physician, 1971; Muus, 1970; Tanner, 1968).

These factors require some elaboration. Thus, since puberty may start anytime from the age of 9 to 16 years, and physical growth may cease at any age between 13 and 20 years, one youth may have completed his physical development when another of the same chronologic age is just beginning. The variation in the speed of growth allows for further discrepancies between subjects of the same chronologic age. The significance of these wide variations between chronologic peers becomes even more impressive when we recall the impact on many youths of the sharp acceleration in physical development (Frazier and Lisonbee, 1950), necessitating as it does acute awareness of the crystallizing identity and rapid (and for a time repeated) modification of the body image (which for many years preceding puberty has remained farily stable and relatively unnoticed, owing to the slow, regular rate of growth up to puberty). Self-consciousness is augmented by late or abnormal development (Clayton et al., 1967; Gallagher, 1966, 1969; Schonfeld, 1950, 1964), by the reactions of adults (particularly parents), to the muscular and sexual blooming during this period (Anthony, 1969), and by the value judgments (in terms of masculinity, femininity, social prestige and athletic prowess) which the peer group and society in general attach to the stage and dimensions of physical development.

The early maturer has advantages over those peers of the same chronologic age whose onset of puberty has been later or whose rate of growth is slower, even though within normal health limits. The early maturer has a higher score on intelligence tests at all ages up to 17, greater athletic competence, is stronger and heavier, usually socially more self-confident, and is endowed by the youth subculture(s) with greater prestige. Adults tend to rate him as "more attractive" and his teacher is more likely to treat him as an equal. Early maturers have been found to gain significantly more success in examinations for entrance to secondary schools, and the reports of teachers on their behavior may also be more favorable than those for late maturers (Tanner, 1962). Girls who have begun to menstruate have been found to score higher on certain psychologic measures of emotional maturity than girls who have yet to start, while in a group of 17-year-old girls given a particular psychologic test, those who were late maturers revealed greater feelings of inadequacy and rejection (Tanner, 1962).

The early maturer does not have everything in his or her favor, however—adults may misconstrue advanced physical maturity as implying more emotional or social maturity than the youth has had time and experience to acquire, and may thus thrust him into positions of responsibility, independence and decision-making which he is not yet able to manage. It is in this context that Erik

Erikson's concept of adolescence as a psychosocial moratorium—a "time-out" during which the youth can organize the various components of his evolving identity—is so useful, cautioning us to give the youth time and opportunity to test and consolidate his emerging abilities, values and interests.

There are, too, some biologic risks for the early maturer; we have noted that the development of muscle strength lags about 1 year behind body growth, and undue exertion or athletic demands can result in injury, especially to the ends of long bones (Medical Post, 1968; Gallagher, 1966). Girls who mature earlier than their chronologic peers tend to have more difficulty with, and less healthy attitudes towards, menstruation. Girls with particularly tall stature have their own particular problems (Gallagher, 1969; Wettenhall and Roche, 1965) as do boys and girls with precocious puberty (Money, 1970; Sigurjonsdottir and Hayles, 1968).

There is a proven trend, for more than the past 100 years, for puberty to occur at a progressively earlier age and for youth to be taller and heavier than those of previous generations (although the latter trend seems to be leveling off in the United States) (Duche et al., 1966; Tanner, 1968). After examining all available data, Tanner (1968) concludes: "The main conclusion is perfectly clear: girls have experienced menarche (the onset of menstruation) progressively earlier during the past 100 years by between three and four months per decade. On this basis puberty is attained $2\frac{1}{2}$ to $3\frac{1}{2}$ years earlier today than it was a century ago." (There is an exception to every rule—the Bundi tribe of New Guinea has no girl menstruating before the age of 17 years). Tanner continues: "The trend in height and weight at the age of puberty is in good agreement with this figure, the 11-year-old children of today having the size of 12-year-olds 30 or 40 years ago." Tanner judges that the earlier puberty trend will continue for another decade or two; Muus (1970) that "if the age of menarche would continue to decline by four months per decade, by 2240 the average four year old would expereince menarche." Though Tanner (1968) judges that the increase in size of youth has been accompanied by "little or no change in overall shape," Garn of the University of Michigan (Muus, 1970), and more recently in the Montreal Star, August 24, 1971, notes that feet and hands are getting bigger, heads longer and faces narrower.

Thus the conflicts of youth (within the individual's own personality, and also between youth and society, including the family) are being met at earlier ages than "when I was your age. . . . . " The social pressures and expectancies of the peer group (and of the communications media) are also being met earlier, without any persuasive evidence of earlier emotional, social or intellectual maturation. At the other end, the period of (at least financial) dependence on parents and various social institutions has been prolonged by the stress (not necessarily wise in view of recent employment difficulties) on the necessity of obtaining an advanced education. The period of youth is thus stretched out, and we are seeing some of the consequences in terms of youth unrest, a more distinct youth subculture, and the like (Dubos, 1969; Muus, 1970; Unwin, 1970). Muus (1970) comments: "Some of the contemporary adolescent problems and conflicts, especially the present concern with the 'generation gap,' may be better understood if one were to consider the earlier biological maturation of youth as contrasted with their chronological age which usually serves as the frame of reference for parents and teachers." The noted microbiologist and geneticist René Dubos (1969) takes note of the trends discussed in the preceding paragraphs and recommends that "the responsibility of natural science is to study the determinants and consequences of these biological and behavioural changes. The role of social and human sciences is to ex-

amine their desirability." The implication, if judged undesirable, is chilling, although modern futurists have been
trying to prepare us for such dilemmas. Dubos made his
comment as part of an address on ethical issues involved
in genetic manipulation and biologic conditioning.

COMMON COMPLICATIONS

Apart from the significance of early and late maturation as discussed above, there are a few conditions so
common during the growth of youth that they bear some
brief mention. These common hazards of youth are too
often treated as trivial, although they can have an impact on body image, self-concept and identity. As an example, we should note that research does not support the
common belief that a period of muscular incoordination
and consequent awkwardness is a frequent normal consequence of the rapid growth of youth—the clumsy youth
is likely to have been a clumsy child.

Acne

This condition (Gallagher, 1966) is too often passed
off by adults as something of little significance, although
most physicians who work with youth have known
young persons who have reacted with exquisite
self-consciousness, depression and even social withdrawal
to protracted or severe attacks of acne. As an editorial in
the British Medical Journal (June 30, 1962, p. 1819) noted:
"It is encouraging that so much attention is being paid to
a problem which, in the past, has too often been treated as
trivial." Certainly, the majority of young people do notice
and are concerned about even small areas of pustules—a
concern which the cosmetics, pharmaceutical and ad-
vertising industries have reinforced and exploited.

Explanation of the nature of the skin changes responsible for the condition, clear advice concerning food

and body hygiene, prescription of appropriate cleansing and drying agents, and an outline of the anticipated course of the complaint can be of inestimable help in reassuring the patient. In general, the pustules will be in evidence particularly between the ages of 13 and 18, clearing first from the face while spreading on the back, then clearing from the back by about the age of 18 or 19. Youths with severe cases should be referred to a dermatologist; plastic surgery may be recommended for the scarring in severe cases, although the youth should be made aware of the uncertain results of such procedures (Epstein, 1968).

Obesity

Obesity is a condition never to be ignored in adolescence, even when there is no associated hormonal or other pathologic condition (Bruch, 1969, 1970; Lorber, 1967; Soloman, 1969). There is a simple form of obesity in youth which often gives rise to concern about hormonal abnormalities and may invite unnecessary specialized investigation. This form occurs particularly just prior to the onset of puberty, or sometimes just before the height spurt of mid-adolescence. In boys, the distribution of fat is such that the silhouette approximates feminine contours, while excessive fat in the pubic area may partly bury a normally developing penis and make it appear under-developed or even infantile. These false impressions of diminished masculinity will be noticed by both the individual and his peers—and the comments of the latter are rarely tactful, at a time when the youth is suddenly acutely aware of the differences between boys and girls. The outcome may be a disturbance of sexual identity, and at the least a miserable early adolescence.

Another type of obesity, related to adolescence, is commonly thought to be due to self-indulgence in the form of overeating. Although such forms of obesity do exist, and require assessment of emotional factors and the advisability of psychotherapy, research indicates that many obese youths in fact eat less than their peers of lighter weight, but undertake far less physical activity. Current therapy for this style of obesity tends to steer away from restrictive diets and to encourage forcefully more exercise.

Breast Enlargement in Boys

A simple form of breast enlargement is present in boys more frequently than we realize. Many boys around the age of 15 have a disc of at least 10-mm diameter under the nipple; it can be felt with the fingers and is tender. This thickening tends to go away spontaneously within a year or two without treatment and does not indicate any abnormal condition. There is no associated abnormality of the sex hormones in the body and no treatment other than reassurance is necessary, although the reassurance does need to be repeated frequently as this condition is regarded with considerable apprehension by many boys.

There is another condition in which the whole breast swells (either one or both breasts may be involved) and attains young feminine contours; again there is no hormonal abnormality, but when the condition does not disappear spontaneously an operation to remove some of the fat may be indicated.

Striae Atrophicae

Striae atrophicae are purplish-pink scar-like depressions in the skin. They are usually associated with pregnancy in women, but can be found in obese people, including young boys (especially between the ages of 11 and 17 years). Apart from disfigurement, their significance, as for obesity and for breast enlargement, lies in the relationship which youth assumes they have to femininity.

EFFECTS OF PSYCHOLOGIC AND SOCIAL FACTORS

In closing, one should refer briefly to the effects which psychologic and social factors can have on physical development. This is an area about which we know only a little, although the classical studies of Rene Spitz and John Bowlby on the effects of emotional deprivation are ample evidence in themselves. The issue is becoming increasingly prominent and pertinent as evidence accumulates on the deleterious effects of poverty, poor housing and general socioeconomic deprivatìon on intellectual, personality and physical development. One of the most fascinating chance findings of the effects of psychologic factors on growth is that reported by Widdowson (1951); despite a special diet and increased food intake, a group of orphans failed, as a result of exposure to a harsh castigating housemother, to achieve the same gain in height and weight as a routinely fed control group. The influence of social background on physical growth was demonstrated by Meredith (1951) who surveyed studies made throughout North America and found that, in mid-childhood, boys reared in poverty were more than 2 inches shorter and 5 pounds lighter than comparable boys of the wealthier classes.

The words of Duche and his co-authors (1966) sum up the intent of this chapter: "the understanding of adolescent personality development and the significance of specific behaviour would be enhanced if the mental health specialists were to correlate their findings not only with the chronological age but also with the level of (physical) development."

REFERENCES

Anthony, J. (1969): The reactions of adults to adolescents and their behavior. In: *Adolescence: Psychosocial Perspectives*. G. Caplan and S. Lebovici (Eds.) Basic Books, Inc., New York.

Bruch, H. (1969): Obesity in adolescence. In: G. Caplan and S. Lebovici., Eds. op. cit.

Bruch, H. (1970): Eating disorders in adolescence. In: *The Psychopathology of Adolescence.* J. Zubin and A. M. Freedman, (Eds.) Grune & Stratton, New York.

Canadian Family Physician (1971): Eskimo growth increase. 17 (2):23.

Chiazze, L., Brayer, F. T., Macisco. J. J., Parker, M. P. and Duffy, B. J. (1968): Length and variability of the menstrual cycle. J.A.M.A., 203:377–380.

Clayton, B. E., Tanner, J. M., Newns, G. H., Whitehouse, R. H. and Renwick, A. G. L. (1967): Differential diagnosis of children with short stature not associated with metabolic, chromosomal or gross nervous system defects. Arch. Dis. Child. 42:245–258.

Donovan, B. T. and Van der Werf Ten Bosch, J. J. (1965): *Physiology of Puberty.* Williams & Wilkins Co., Baltimore.

Dubos, R. (1969): Ethical issues involved in genetic manipulation and biologic conditioning. In: *The Ethics of Change.* Toronto, Canadian Broadcasting Corporation Publications, p. 21.

Duche, D. J., Schonfeld, W. A. and Tomkiewicz, S. (1966): Physical aspects of adolescent development. In: *Psychiatric Approaches to Adolescence.* G. Caplan and S. Lebovici (Eds.) Excerpta Medica, Amsterdam.

Epstein, E. (1968): Present status of dermabrasion. J.A.M.A. 206: 607–610.

Frazier, A. and Lisonbee, L. K. (1950): Adolescent concerns with physique. School Review 58:397–405.

Gallagher, J. R. (1966): *Medical Care of the Adolescent.* Appleton-Century-Crofts, New York.

Gallagher, J. R. (1969): Short and tall stature in otherwise normal adolescents: management of their medical and psychologic problems. In: *Endocrine and Genetic Diseases of Childhood,* L. I. Gardener (Ed.) W. B. Saunders Co., Philadelphia.

Gardener, L. I. (1960): Biochemical events at adolescence. Pediat. Clin. N. Amer. 7:15–31.

Garell, D. C. (1968): Sex education—an adolescent clinic responsibility. Adolescent Medicine Newsletter 4 (2):2–10.

Johanson, A. J., Guyda, H., Light, C., Migeon, C. and Blizzard, R. (1969): Serum luteinizing hormone by radio-immunoassay in normal children. J. Pediat. 74:416–424.

Kestenberg, J. S. (1967): Phases of adolescence: with suggestions for a correlation of psychic and hormonal organization. J. Amer. Acad. Child Psychiat. 6:426–463.

King, A. (1966): Venereal disease problems and adolescent health. Clin. Pediat. 5:597–603.

Kirkendall, L. A. and Calderwood, D. (1965): *Selected References on Sex Education*. American Academy of Pediatrics, Chicago.

Lelong, M. et al. (1957): Une enquête sur la croissance des garçons francais. Sem. Hop. Paris (Ann. Pediat.) 33:2721–2724.

Levy, D. M. (1929): A method for integrating physical and psychiatric examination. Amer. J. Psychiat. 9:121–194.

Lorber, J. (1967): Obesity in childhood. Clin. Pediat. 6:325–326.

Medical Post (1968): Childhood athletics new suspect in hip osteoarthritis. Feb. 27, p. 8.

Meredith, H. V. (1951): Relation between socioeconomic status and body size in boys seven to ten years of age. Amer. J. Dis. Child. 82:702–709.

Money, J. (1970): Hormonal and genetic extremes at puberty. In: J. Zubin and A. M. Freedman (Eds.) op. cit.

Muus, R. E. (1970): Adolescent development and the secular trend. Adolescence 5:267–284.

Nellhaus, G. (1968): Head circumference: birth to 18 years. Pediatrics 41:106–114.

Osofosky, H. J. (1968): *The Pregnant Teenager: A Medical, Educational and Social Analysis*. Charles C Thomas, Springfield, Ill.

Reynolds, E. L. and Wines, J. V. (1948): Individual differences in physical changes associated with adolescence in girls. Amer. J. Dis. Child. 75:329–350.

Reynolds, E. L. and Wines, J. V. (1951): Physical changes associated with adolescence in boys. Amer. J. Dis. Child. 82:529–547.

Schonfeld, W. A. (1950): Inadequate masculine physique. Psychosom. Med. 12:49–54.

Schonfeld, W. A. (1964): Body image disturbances in adolescents with inappropriate sexual development. Amer. J. Orthopsychiat. 35:493–502.

Schonfeld, W. A. (1969): The body and the body-image in adolescents. In: G. Caplan and S. Lebovici (Eds.) op. cit.

Schulz, E. D. and Williams, S. R. (1969): *Family Life and Sex Education. Curriculum and Instruction*. Harcourt, Brace and World, New York.

Sigurjonsdottir, T. J. and Hayles, A. B. (1968): Precocious puberty. Amer. J. Dis. Child. 115:309–322.

Solomon, N. (1969): The study and treatment of the obese patient. Hosp. Practice 4:90–94.

Stuart, H. C. (1946): Normal growth and development during adolescence. New Eng. J. Med. 234:666–672, 693–700, 732–738.

Tanner, J. M. (1962): *Growth at Adolescence.* Blackwell Scientific Publications, Oxford.

Tanner, J. M. (1968): Earlier maturation in man. Sci. Amer. 218:21–27.

Unwin, J. R. (1968): Somatic development in adolescence. Canad. Family Physician, 14(10):33–38.

Unwin, J. R. (1970): Perspectives on contemporary youth. Canad. Family Physician 16(6):47–53.

Weldon, V. V., Kowarski, A. and Migeon, C. J. (1967): Aldosterone secretion rates in normal subjects from infancy to adulthood. Pediatrics 39:713–723.

Wettenhall, H. N. B. and Roche, A. F. (1965): Tall girls: assessment and management. Aust. Paediatric J. 1:219–226.

Widdowson, E. M. (1951): Mental contentment and physical growth. Lancet 1:1316–1318.

World Health Organization (1965): Health Problems of Adolescence: *Report of a WHO Expert Committee.* Techn. Rep. Ser., p. 308.

Yen, S. S. C., Vicic, W. J. and Kearchner, D. V.: Gonadotropin levels in puberty. J. Clin. Endocr. 29:382–385.

Young, H. B. et al.(1968): Evaluation of physical maturity at adolescence. Develop. Med. Child Neurol. 10:338–348.

Zacharias, L. and Wurtman, R. J. (1969): Age at menarche: genetic and environmental influences. New Eng. J. Med., 280:868–875.

Chapter 4

SOME IMPLICATIONS OF THE SEXUAL REVOLUTION FOR YOUTH

James F. Masterson, Jr.

Sexual mores are changing. Mankind is undergoing yet another dramatic swing of the pendulum in his effort to integrate harmoniously his sexual impulses and his social values. The evidence is everywhere: Newspapers report that students insist that sex is a private matter and demand the right to entertain girls in their rooms. The pill, which can mean only one pill, is more and more widely used. The abortion rate is rising while the percentage of those who have not had sexual intercourse prior to marriage is falling. The ancient fears of disapproval, of disease, of death and of damnation are losing their former sway. Are these changes only in attitude or are they also manifested in behavior? Are they the views and actions of a prophetic minority, the wave of the future, or rather of a fringe group, licentious and rebellious? Is this revolution or evolution? Will it lead to a decline in social morality or to greater human happiness? Is it only among the young, or does the older generation also participate? Why is it happening now? This chapter, presenting some reflections on these questions, also describes some of the implications of these changes for the adolescent's struggle to develop sexual identity.

Many of us elders, viewing these changes from the perspective of our own development (one based for the most part on Judeo-Christian ethics and strict concepts of sexual morality), have tended to see them as a "sexual revolution" and to ascribe them primarily to youth. It seems to me that we may err on both counts for not only is this ferment taking place among adults, but also, what we call revolution—meaning the overthrow of an established system of morals the younger generation may view as evolution—meaning the process of growth and development toward a new system of morals.

Let us examine first the adult world for evidence of change. This evidence has been accumulating so rapidly that as I was preparing this paper I found myself constantly changing my examples as new evidence flooded in. I finally resolved the problem by limiting the examples to three social institutions, i.e., religion, law and medicine.

The recent deliberations of the ecumenical council called by Pope John brought about some changes in Catholic thinking about sex. This is perhaps as it should be, since the Catholic Church has been more responsible than any other single agency for the prevailing concepts of sexual morality that have guided Western Man for the last 2000 years. Many aspects of sexual morality were dealt with at Vatican Council II, but I would like to mention only two, i.e., those relating to the purpose of sexual intercourse and to birth control. The Church had previously emphasized that the sole purpose of sexual intercourse was to have children and thereby propagate the faithful. Yielding to the pressures caused by the findings of depth psychology, the Church has begun to consider broadening its views to include the promotion of marital harmony as an equally valid purpose of sexual intercourse. My second example, the deliberations on birth control, received such widespread publicity that I need only mention that this hot coal so threatened to divide he Council that it was referred to the Pope who, despite the opinion of his advisory board, does not know what to do. If he follows the recommendation of the advisory board and liberalizes the church's views on birth control he will offend the conservatives. If he doesn't, the laity may rebel as some already have. So this ancient and venerable institution is now in conflict over its view of sex.

Second, let us turn to the law. There is great agitation throughout the country to liberalize abortion laws. A recent survey of psychiatrists indicated that 95 percent felt the laws should be liberalized. Efforts to achieve this end failed in New York State in 1971, but they succeeded in Colorado. To cite another example, a bill was submitted to the English Parliament making homosexual acts between consenting adults not a crime. Thus, the law also is revising its views on the handling of sexual matters.

Finally in medicine, for the first time in the history of mankind the light of reason in the form of experimental scientific study has been introduced into the darkness, superstition and mystery that have surrounded human sexuality by Masters and Johnson's unique and pioneering study of human sexual behavior.

These changes in the Catholic Church, in the law, and in medicine cannot be ascribed only to youth. Clearly the older generation, those charged with preserving, protecting and transmitting the values of our culture, are actively involved in modifying these very same values.

What is happening among younger people? While thier elders, being under less immediate pressure from sexual feelings cope with these issues in a sober and intellectual fashion, the young people of today, under more urgent pressure, have leapfrogged their parents to apply these newer concepts to their own lives. Authorities differ as to the extent of premarital intercourse amongst students, but there is consensus that the double standard increasingly is being discarded, that college girls more often seek sexual experience during the college years than their mothers did. There is evidence of earlier biologic maturation in adolescence, a widespread pattern of going steady, and of more open and vocal discussion of sex.

How extensive is this change? Although I read much in in the press about the increased sexual freedom of the younger generation, I see less of this in my office and read even less about it in professional publications. I think our fears about sexual misbehavior have led us to underrate the fact that beginning sexual experience for many youngsters is often frought with anguish and pain, and, therefore, can be as much a trial as a pleasure. One does not remove, as easily as an overcoat, values which, transmitted from generation to generation, have been inculcated into one's conscience throughout childhood. This takes time and testing and trial—i.e., evolution not revolution—both at the social level and the individual level. My guess is that the advanced guard of the younger generation is indeed exhibiting a great deal more sexual freedom but that the majority, while still holding to traditional patterns in their behavior even as their parents did, are at the same time submitting their concepts, previously taken for granted, to serious and searching scrutiny. In other words, there is more change in attitude than in behavior. This view was supported recently by Halleck (1967) who found, in his survey of girls at The University of Wisconsin, that although 70 percent thought there was nothing wrong with premarital sexual intercourse, only 22 percent actually engaged in it.

I see more actual sexual freedom among those in their

mid-20's, who have passed their adolescent phase of sexual development and have a more secure sexual identity. Among these, traditional sexual morality has given way to the following view: Sexual play is avoided, if possible, unless the boy and girl care about each other. When they do care, sexual play occurs as a preliminary to sexual intercourse, which itself is seen as important, but subordinate to a higher value, i.e., a close interpersonal relationship. They have replaced the ancient virtue of chastity with that of fidelity, meaning that a girl has no compunctions about having sexual intercourse with a boy with whom she is in love, but today would no more think of being promiscuous than her mother did 20 years ago, but for entirely different reasons. The following excerpt from *Group for Advancement of Psychiatry* (1965) provides an example.

Sally was an especially gifted student, interested in her work, and gave promise of a successful creative career. In high school, she had had her eye on getting into a good college. She had not been active in the social life of school, which seemed to her superficial. In her freshman year at college, she threw herself into a whirl of active dating, received many invitations, and was very popular. When she had satisfied herself that she was desirable and could carry off social occasions well, some of the excitement of dating began to pall and she sought more meaningful relationships. She now dated only boys with whom she felt she could establish a deeper emotional and intellectual relationship. One of the boys she came to know better wanted to have sexual relations. She described her reaction: "For me it is a special thing. I am sort of monogamous. I don't like to diffuse to a lot of people. I like to have close friends even though I know a lot of people. As far as I am concerned, intercourse is one thing where you are giving a lot of yourself to one person. I never wanted to do it unless I was absolutely sure about that person and I never was; particularly when I started realizing that these people did not care much about my welfare or about me as a person. It impressed me as if they almost had to prove to themselves and also to other people that they could do it. It was a competitive thing."

Sally had not expected to engage in sexual relations in college. In her junior year, however, she met a boy who, she said, was "interested in my interests and I was interested in his interests." Eventually, they had intercourse. Here is her description of her feelings: "It got to the point where it really got frustrating not doing it. We had been going out together seven or eight months and it seemed—if you feel strongly about a person and if you really love him—I don't see anything really wrong about it, because it is a complete relationship, as complete as for some people who get married. This is one action where you give everything you have to the other person. There is always a circumstance of holding back and it would have been wrong; it would have been almost wrong to keep holding back something that I really wanted to give him."

To those who would be alarmed that this sort of change may lead to a decline in morality, I would suggest that we are not seeing orgies or lack of control, but rather a different kind of control—self-control based not on guilt, or fear of disapproval, but on a concept of human relations that emphasizes self-respect, human worth and human dignity.

What are the reasons for this change? Perhaps we might get some insight by considering first how the standards that are undergoing change arose in the first place. Let us journey back in time for a moment to that critical period for the development of Western civilization —Rome around the first century A.D. Prior to that time, during the expansion of the Roman Empire, sexual standards had been strict and social morality was quite high and conducive to the strength of the society and the growth of the Roman Republic. However, Rome's new-found affluence, power and leisure led to a deterioration of sexual standards. The Emperor, worried about the future of his realm, between 18 and 9 B.C., promulgated a series of laws which have been called the most important social legislation of antiquity. A crucial law for the first time forbade a husband to kill an adulteress wife and ordered him under severe fines to bring her to court and accuse her. That which had been a private wrong became the state's business for the first time. A whole series of laws were promulgated in an effort to prop up the birth rate of the upper classes, e.g., bachelors, spinsters and childless wives were ineligible to inherit; mothers of three or more children were given special legal privileges; political preference between equal candidates was given to the man who had the greater number of children. However, to a more or less degree, every one of these laws was a failure. Roman philosophers began to argue in favor of sexual restraint and even asceticism. Now where legislation and law had failed religion succeeded. Christian morality allied itself to these latter forces and effectively displaced the traditional Greco-Roman patterns of sexuality and began a new concept of sexual morality which survives until this day. It emphasized chastity, virginity, and the spiritual merit of denying the flesh. It is these very standards which originated 2000 years ago that are under challenge today. Is it not possible that these standards which have served so well for so many years may at the same time contain some inherent handicaps to human self-expression which the younger generation are no longer willing to accept? And, therefore, may they not view their efforts to emancipate themselves from their heritage as evolutionary rather than revolutionary?

A second contributive cause is the decreasing impact of religion and the increasing impact of science in our daily lives. The profound discoveries of modern science have so lessened our dependence on the forces of nature, that they have led to an emphasis on the use of reason rather than religion in the conduct of one's life. There has been a corresponding waning of the influence of religion as reflected in the discussions of the "God is Dead" theory. This has caused adolescents today, more than in earlier times, to demand logical reasons for ethical standards. It no longer suffices to speak to them of what is right and wrong in terms of some kind of natural moral law.

A third cause has been the pervasive influence of the psychoanalytic view that the failure to integrate sexual impulses and feelings into the personality in a healthy way impairs personality growth and produces emotional difficulties.

A fourth cause is the increasingly strong demands of women for equality on all levels. Women perceive the double standard as keeping them from enjoying the pleasures of love-making which men enjoy without serious social condemnation. This rebellion is not in the direction of curbing men but rather towards releasing women. Finally, the development of the pill, which has freed womankind from its ancient servitude to pregnancy, and the efficacy of penicillin, which has minimized the danger of infection, have removed two common sources of both sexual anxiety and control.

You might well ask at this point what does all this have to do with the adolescent's sexual problems? The adolescent's older brother and sister are carrying out the revolution but he is the one who must come to grips with its effects, for he develops his sexual identity through inter- action with his fellows and with the sexual mores of his culture. Therefore, he is confronted with the shifting sands of a changing sexual morality in the social sphere at a time in his life when lacking a personal sense of sexual identity, he must wade through those shifting sands in order to find that identity. Although the unstable social climate immeasurably complicates his development, since it gives him few certainties upon which to rest, at the same time it may afford him a greater potential by giving him more freedom to experiment to find that identity. The question is pertinent here as to how easy it has ever been in our culture for an adolescent to learn healthy sexual attitudes. Unless he has been fortunate enough to learn it from his parents where can he find out? From watching a James Bond movie, or reading books like "The Carpetbaggers," from such voyeuristic notions as the Playboy Club, or from the melange of neurotic attitudes towards sex presented on the Broadway stage?

What are some of the implications of this revolution? Let us consider the benefits first and then the hazards. There are many adolescents who, immature or excessively inhibited, come to a dangerously late period of their development before fully realizing that they have sexual problems. The revolution may impel these to recognize and seek help for their problem earlier. For example:

Jean, a 22-year-old senior at one of the better eastern girls' colleges, sat in my office and hesitantly and tearfully told the following story: She had always been popular with boys since she began dating at 14. Initially she had reveled in her success as proof of her femininity, but when she first became involved with a boy at 16 she developed such severe anxiety, nausea and vomiting on each date that her only recourse was to end the relationship. She allayed her doubts with the thought that she would grow out of this difficulty but time was to prove her wrong. The pattern was already set and it continued unabated through the next 6 years. She feels she must have dated at least 100 boys in college and everytime one became close the symptoms would resume and she would have to break off. She had to settle for an endless round of superficial dating without daring to have a close relationship with a boy. I could not help wondering as I listened to this attractive but immature girl that more pressure of the kind implied by the sex revolution might have brought her for help sooner.

Another example:

> A 19-year-old girl, a college sophomore, had been having emotional difficulties since the onset of puberty when she became anxious, depressed, withdrew from her friends, and spent all of her time on school work. It was necessary for the parents to send her away to a special school for treatment. Gradually she improved, finished high school, and entered college, where she again became anxious and depressed and came to my office for treatment. Although she maintained an active social life with an average amount of dating she had never had a close relationship with a boy nor had she experienced any sexual activity—neither of which was a source of concern to her. After a year of intensive treatment and much "working through" of her anxiety and depression it became clear that she was so terrified of sexual feelings and impulses that she avoided any occasion with boys that might provoke them. She had always been dimly aware, without facing up to the fact, that something was wrong with her and, again without facing the fact, anticipated that she would grow up to be an "old maid." The summer of her freshman year she took a cross-country trip with some girl friends and was amazed to find on visiting a number of campuses throughout the midwest and the west that girls her age were living with boys. This confrontation with changing sex standards brought home to her in a profound way her own sexual immaturity and motivated her to work on her sexual difficulties through treatment. Twenty years ago this girl's sexual difficulty may well have escaped notice, perhaps even up to marriage.

What about the hazards? The sexual revolution may precipitate a premature attempt at sexual relations either by those who are immature and not ready for it or by those who, overinhibited, cannot accept the emotional consequences of their actions. Efforts then become abortive and can have disastrous consequences for emotional life as suggested by the following case:

An 18-year-old freshman in college, who came from a well-to-do Puerto Rican family, was raised as a strict Catholic, and attended private Catholic schools. His father, feeling no further religious guidance was necessary, encourage the youth to attend an Ivy League school. Here he came, for the first time, under the influence of differing views about sexual behavior, and when he fell in love with a girl from another eastern college he would rendezvous with her in a New York hotel bedroom where they would spend the afternoon lying in bed necking. Driven by his impulses, but unable to consummate them because of his conscience, he developed intolerable sexual tension which he later relieved by masturbation which led to depression and feelings of inadequacy. In these depressions he would roam the streets of New York all night seeking solace. Overwhelmed by these feelings, he finally was unable to do his school work, dropped out of college and was referred for treatment. It took many months for him to understand the conflict between his sexual impulses and his standards.

At this point a few thoughts about management of sexual problems may be in order. Too often, we abandon our youngsters at this crucial time of life to work out their sexual problems by themselves. We afford them no easy channels of communication to check their thoughts and impulses without being criticized or reprimanded. I suspect we do this because, often as not, the emergence of their sexuality recalls to us the sexual problems which we encountered at that time of life and which we have spent a good many years trying to repress. So, first and foremost, the physician should be aware of the degree of comfort that he feels in talking about sex, and if he is uncomfortable it would be better for him to refer his patient to another physician.

To those who do wish to help these youngsters, it may be of some interest to learn how the psychiatrist goes about it. The psychiatrist views sexual behavior as a component part of the total personality, and attempts to understand the sexual problem as one bit of evidence that the total personality may be emotionally disturbed. For example, the same sexual act can have an entirely different meaning if performed by a frightened immature dependent girl to gain favor than if performed by a hardened psychopath to relieve sexual tension. In other words, the psychiatrist evaluates a sexual problem as he would any other symptom—in the total context of the personality and the situation. Does the problem represent an isolated incident or a pattern? Does it represent an effort to relieve anxiety and depression, as seems to be the case with most of my patients, or is it an appropriate attempt to experiment and find sexual identity? Is it conducive to or harmful to personality development? Or does it represent a more serious underlying pathologic condition such as a perversion? The psychiatrist must be alert to those who are inhibited and immature, for the consequences for their future sexual life can be as serious as for those with a more obvious pathologic condition. He investigates the childhood background to see how the behavior fits with the conscience as developed through childhood.

How does the psychiatrist act, once he thinks he understands? As always, in accord with the best interests of the patient. If the patient's behavior is not harmful to himself or others, he may reassure or encourage him. If it is harmful, he confronts the patient with the fact. He neither lectures nor admonishes, but seeks to help the patient understand the ramifications of his problem. He discusses directly and openly both the developmental and the social issues raised by the patient's behavior. He might suggest that sexual life has to be subordinated to the total personality and its well-being as well as to human relationships, and that it therefore entails responsibility in addition to the pursuit of pleasure. Indeed, the greatest pleasure can be found when it is subordinated in this way. And, finally, he keeps in mind that the goal of his efforts is to keep his patient's developmental pathway open to a healthy and mature adult sexual life—one that combines the utmost in pleasure with the necessary amount of responsibility first to the patient's own conscience, and then to his fellow human beings.

REFERENCES

Group for the Advancement of Psychiatry (1965): *Sex and the College Student,* Report #60. Mental Health Materials Center, Inc., New York, pp. 38–39.

Halleck, S. (1967): Sex and mental health on the campus. J.A.M.A. 200(8):684–689.

Section II

CLINICAL PROBLEMS AND
TREATMENT APPROACHES

Chapter 5

YOUTH AND MENTAL HEALTH: AN INTERVIEW WITH IRENE JOSSELYN

Irene Josselyn practices in Phoenix, Arizona. She has been helping and treating young people for the past three decades. Besides having a certification in child psychiatry she is a qualified psychiatric social worker and a trained psychoanalyst.

Her interest in problems of disturbed youth started at an early age, her father, Orris Milliken, was a pioneer in helping delinquent adolescents and she grew up learning principles of child guidance.

With clinical experience gained over many years she sees the strengths and the weaknesses of contemporary youth, and relates it to bringing-up patterns. She looks at the influence psychoanalysis has had in changing those patterns. She describes the differences in youth coming for help today and those who came three decades ago. With an insight and understanding which can only come from years of helping and listening to youth, she provides guidelines and warns of pitfalls for any one who undertakes the difficult but rewarding task of helping an emotionally disturbed adolescent.

Question: Most adolescents are referred because of behavior problems such as stealing, truancy and promiscuity. Do you feel that it is useful to categorize adolescents with such emotional problems diagnostically? Do you also think that there is a classification which is satisfactory?

Irene Josselyn: Once you rule out the psychosis and a typical severe neurosis, which I feel we should not put into the category of adolescence but rather in a category of the specific diagnosis, the only diagnosis we need is "adolescence."

It is important to define how I am using the term "adolescence." I do not see it as a chronologic age; I see it as a step in psychologic maturation. It is a fluid state because many childhood conflicts are revisited and there is a struggle to attain an adult identity. This is the diagnostic definition that I would use in dealing with the adolescent. I feel that if we try to break it down into more delineated classifications, we get into the danger of losing our own fluidity in understanding the adolescent. Any diagnostic differentiation that I have seen, except for the severe neurosis and the psychoses, implies an evaluation of the origin and permanency of the condition.

I don't think the average adolescent who comes to us with manifest problems will necessarily show the same problem tomorrow. The problems change. This to me is the diagnosis of psychologic adolescence. Certain chronologically so-called adolescents, I feel, are not adolescents. Some are still children. Others, I feel, have become crystallized into an adult neurosis and the dynamics then is the same as with any adult neurosis. So in diagnosis I would prefer the broad term "adolescence" rather than anything more specific.

Question: If I understand you rightly, you are saying that if one sees an adolescent whose primary psychopathology appears to be impulsivity, to diagnose him as an impulsive adolescent might hamper treatment because this adolescent may be impulsive today and move into being nonimpulsive tomorrow, yet remain a behavior-problem adolescent.

Irene Josselyn: Most typical adolescents are, at time, impulsive. You may find that their impulsiveness today is counteracted or is in contrast to the compulsive element in their personality as you get to know them better. As another example of this, if we say that the individual is asocial, what do we mean? We are describing what society is objecting to, but not what is going on within him. We need to know what is going on within him rather than put it in terms of social condemnation.

Question: Following what you just said, you don't seem to think that breaking down these behavior disorders in adolescence into diagnostic categories is of any help in terms of charting out the treatment and management.

Irene
Josselyn:
I say this because I feel that when you chart out the treatment you lose your flexibility in treatment. We have to make a diagnosis for insurance companies, but I think that the more we can evaluate the behavior as "adolescence," and deal with it as such, the better. This excludes that group that belongs in a fixed category, since I don't think that most of our adolescents, except the severely disturbed, fit into a fixed category.

In the example you gave, you make a diagnosis, after you have seen the adolescent once or twice, of an impulsive character. Then 3 or 4 weeks later you begin to see signs that his impulsiveness doesn't fit every place, so you say, "Boy, I'm really successful, I've cured an impulsive character." I don't think that you were necessarily successful at all. What you have seen is the other side of the coin of this fluid adolescent.

In another instance you may make a diagnosis of an inability to relate to another person, a narcissistic picture; 4 or 5 weeks later you find out that the adolescent really has formed a very positive feeling for you. So you say, "I am a successful therapist; here I am converting a narcissistic personality into a person capable of loving." But he probably was capable of loving when you made a diagnosis of narcissistic character; he just hadn't reached the point that he loved you yet, and was not revealing his readiness to relate. This is what is so hard with treating the adolescent, in contrast to working with children or adults. We don't have the clues to really make a true diagnosis because the clues aren't there; it is too confused a picture for us.

Question: You have been in the field of adolescent psychiatry longer than anybody else I know in North America. Do you see any change in the type of picture the adolescent is presenting in terms of his clinical manifestation today from what you saw 20 years ago?

Irene Josselyn: Yes, I have been trying to think when I saw the change and I would say that about 10 or 15 years ago I began to see a change which I didn't recognize until recently.

I have a feeling that the adolescent of today is less emotionally prepared for the problems of adolescence than any I have ever seen before. In other words, I am seeing a group of adolescents who are showing emotional problems that, from my past experience, I would expect them to handle better. I am seeing a group who have been brought up in a child-centered world (this is by no means a general characterization of all adolescents), who still believe they have a right to be in a child-centered world. This is a group with whom I feel we have really failed because we didn't prepare them for adolescence. I am really surprised at the number of adolescents who do not show this in view of our theory of child-rearing in a child-centered world.

I see three categories where I feel this is significant. I see the adolescent who believes he has a right to everything. This attitude has always been true of adolescents to a certain extent, but I have never seen it to such a degree as I am seeing it now. I see a group of adolescents who have a longing for closeness that earlier I saw only in adolescents who either had a very deprived childhood, or who had acted in a way to alienate people. Now I observe this longing for closeness in those who come from "the best kind of childhood." Thirdly, I am seeing a group of adolescents who are creative, intelligent, imaginative, but who are not seeing their adolescence as a challenge but rather as something they can't take.

This is where drugs come in. One aspect of drugs is an escape from challenge. The adolescent experiences no gratification from meeting a challenge. This I believe is part of our child-centered world—that we have overprotected children. Because we knew the psychologically sick child had to be protected, we have assumed that every child needs that kind of protection. I don't think they do. We have a group of adolescents now who should have real confidence in the future that they can create; they don't have this confidence. We have always seen a group with this attitude, but now I am seeing it in young people whom I would expect to be excited about the challenge—they are not; they are defeated by it. Many people defend their attitude by blaming the atomic bomb—no wonder they are discouraged, they may be dead tomorrow from the bomb! Our young people have always faced the danger of their destruction. There have been droughts, there has been the plague, there have been many things which couldn't be prevented. Before we knew something about medicine we couldn't prevent a plague. There is a way to prevent the use of the atomic bomb, but instead of saying, "We will work hard to prevent the use of the atomic bomb," they say, "Oh, what's the use, we are going to be destroyed by the bomb anyway."

Question: Are you saying that the adolescents you are seeing today are emotionally less mature than the adolescents you were seeing 10 or 15 years ago?

Irene Josselyn: No, I don't think it is really immaturity. I would put it rather on the basis that they have fewer tools with which to mature. I don't think they are any less immature, in fact some of them are more mature, if you use just maturation, than those of their age in the past. It's more that they are emotionally ill-equipped to deal with the problems that the adolescent faces.

Question: What would you ascribe that to?

Irene Josselyn: It is partly due to our whole theory of the child-centered world, that is, a child must not be frustrated; a child should be happy. We didn't give him a feeling of challenge. There's another aspect which would take a long dissertation. We have stressed the need of the small child to be loved; we have not recognized the inherent need of an infant to love. As a consequence we have really failed to encourage his very early capacity to love. It has been assumed that his need for love will be converted into a capacity to love. I believe this is false. His being loved contributes to a capacity to love, but I believe there is also an inherent need to love. To give an example, if a child today breaks a toy the child cries, the parent says, "Don't cry dear, I'll buy you another one." They are saying in effect, "You don't have to love the toy, it will come to you without loving it." We deprive the child of mourning if you want to call it that, in our constant attempt to keep the child from being frustrated.

Question: This avoidance of allowing the child to experience frustration, wouldn't you say that this has been largely influenced by psychoanalytical thought?

Irene Josselyn: Psychoanalysis probably aroused guilt in parents, but maybe psychoanalysis was a reflection of the times in answer to the guilt parents were already feeling. I would hate to feel that analysis is responsible for all of our problems today, but I do think that psychoanalysis has put the emphasis on the need to be loved rather than on the inherent need to love.

You see the sort of thing that I have in mind is that we say that the need to love has its origin in the dependency state of the newborn in that he has to be loved to survive—this becomes the anlage (hereditary predisposition) of the later psychologic capacity to accept being loved and to seek being loved. We have overlooked the fact that the newborn infant turns outward biologically for gratification. The rooting reflex perhaps is the most clear-cut example; he seeks the breast, he doesn't lie passively and get the breast. Now this to me is the anlage of an ultimate capacity to love, just as the biologic dependency is the anlage of the need for love and wish to be loved.

The infant also wants to love. When the infant smiles at the parent, one gets the feeling of a real warm interchange. That's not only because the parent has given—it's because the child is giving. When you observe a 6-month-old baby getting pleasure from touching his mother's cheek, it is not only because he feels secure with the mother, but because he gets pleasure out of this contact of giving to the mother as well as receiving from the mother. In our child-rearing, we have ignored this need and therefore failed to develop ideas as to how to foster the child's inherent need to love someone, not just his inherent need to be loved by someone.

Question: From what you have said, I would think you would consider it important to bring the parents into the treatment situation when one is treating the adolescent.

Irene Josselyn: Well, I think it depends on what you mean by bringing them in. I myself have never been very enthusiastic about a continual family therapy with the adolescent unless the primary problem is a superficial one of family relationships.

The reason I say this is because the adolescent has a right to his secrets and I don't like to see an adolescent overexposed by too much knowledge on the part of anyone. One of the values of our relationship with the adolescent is that he can have secrets with us that never go beyond us. On the other hand, I don't know if there are many instances in adolescent therapy in which I would want to have no relationship with the parents.

I found, for example, that if I say to the adolescent, when he brings up some problem, "Now this is a practical problem; I agree with you, your parents don't understand it but you don't understand their point of view and I don't either—let me talk it over with them." Then I tell him what I am going to say. I never violate an adolescent's confidences. When I talk to the parents, sometimes I do it in the presence of the adolescent, and sometimes he prefers not to be present and I accept that.

I try to get the parents to see in broad terms some of the problems of the adolescent—nothing that is confidential to the particular adolescent—and try to get them to see the practical ways that they can help him through this period. Interestingly enough, I have never had an adolescent refuse to let me talk to his parents. As long as he knows that I am going to deal with the parents by explaining his problem to them in general terms, and make suggestions for specific things to try, then he is agreeable to it.

Question: You don't feel that there is any chance that the adolescent will lose trust in the therapist if he knows that the therapist is having a session with his parents alone?

Irene Josselyn: I don't think that the adolescent will lose trust in you if you are trustworthy. By this I mean that if you say something to the parents that appears to the adolescent to be a violation of confidence, then you deserve to lose his trust. In actuality I believe that a session with the parents in which his confidence is not violated will increase his confidence in you.

I realize that there are certain areas where you can get onto very ticklish grounds—for instance, with delinquents. If you know that an adolescent is involved in delinquent behavior that is dangerous you sometimes get into a spot with your own super-ego standards; you will be disloyal to the adolescent if you let this go on. At that point, I am very frank with the adolescent about his behavior. I will say to him, to take an extreme example, "You know that this has got to be stopped. If you continue to act out you are going to be in trouble; I would rather be the one who takes the initiative in working this out rather than having you picked up by the police." The adolescent then knows where I stand. I rarely use this approach though; actually it is one that I used more often in my practice in Chicago where I worked with more delinquents than I do now. However, I think that there are times when one must take this stand and carry it through. It is a risky business, but I don't think that the delinquent adolescent is going to be helped otherwise. By going along with him you are not helping him. You hope that you can direct the consequences so that they will be constructive.

Question: As you say, it is a very risky business, and there will always be the risk that one might lose the adolescent; he might not come for the next interview.

Irene Josselyn: It is possible that you didn't have him to begin with. I wouldn't use this approach in minor things, only in those that are major. If you risk losing him that way you probably didn't have him to begin with, and you are never going to have him. He is going to use you as an excuse for his misbehavior.

Question: How would one avoid, in the treatment of an antisocial acting-out adolescent, one's own super-ego principles? Should one take a very neutral attitude or should one say to the adolescent, "In my opinion what you are doing is dangerous to yourself and dangerous to society"?

Irene Josselyn: You know that this touches on this whole question of value system in psychiatry. I don't believe that any psychiatrist who has any value system fails to convey the value system to his patient no matter how he does it. This idea of our being a blank screen with no standards as far as our adult patients are concerned is a defensive interpretation on our part. The patients know what we stand for. But I think this is particularly important with adolescents because their value system is so confused.

If a patient planned to commit a murder I would naturally tell him he shouldn't do it. If the act is a less asocial one—one in which there is no absolute consensus, but one in which I have value concepts by my philosophy—I'm very honest with him. I say, "You know my own feeling is that this is unwise, for this and that reason." I very carefully explain my reasons, then I imply *and mean it* that he has to work out his own value system. If it is something that is really dangerous for him, then I take a definite stand and perhaps say, "This is dangerous, I don't approve of it; you've got to come to terms with your own feeling about it but know that I'm not supporting it."

A simple example concerns marijuana, the use of which I happen to feel probably should be legalized; however, its use is illegal in this country. I say to my adolescents, "There are several reasons that I don't understand yet why you are using marijuana; we will go into those," but I make it very clear to them that its use is illegal. I will not report them, but I will not defend them if they are caught. As far as I'm concerned what is legal is something that is respected. I've had adolescents say to me, "O.K., don't you ever speed?" and I say, "Yes, but if I am fined for speeding, I pay the fine. I know I was worng. I may disagree with the speed law, I may feel that I should be able to drive faster, but I know what the speed law is and if I violate it, it's not a psychiatric problem, it's a legal problem."

This is the stand that I take on something like marijuana. I don't give the adolescent the feeling that I think it's fine that he smokes marijuana and that if he gets into trouble I will try to get him out of it. I'd be perfectly willing to explain to the court why he uses marijuana if he wants me to and if I know, but I won't ask the court to ignore the legal aspects.

My feeling is that it matters how you tell the adolescent that you disagree with what he is doing, and whether or not you become identified with a parent. I would not say to an adolescent, "I forbid you to do this; you're bad to do it." What I do say to him in effect is, "It seems to me that you are unwise in what you are doing."

Take a very simple example of a junior-high-school kid with a high I.Q., who has plenty of money and can go to college and graduate school if he wants to, who gets angry at the school system and wants to be a drop-out. I point out to him that I think he is foolish, explain why I think he is foolish, and why I think that some of the things he is objecting to could be lived with. I'm saying to him in effect; "My value system is such that you should go to college and you shouldn't drop out of high school." I'm not saying, "You are bad to drop out of high school"; I'm saying, "I respect you enough to give you my thinking on the wisdom of not dropping out of school."

I have said to adolescents on LSD, "Personally I think you are a damned fool. For this and that reason you want to use LSD, and you don't realize the danger you are running into in using it. I just think your judgment is unsound." I'm not saying as a parent would say, if he were destructive in his handling of the situation, "You are a bad boy for using it"; I am expressing very clearly my own value system, explaining why and, in doing so, indicating that I have enough respect for him that I believe that he can think this through. This creates a very different atmosphere from that which most parents create.

Question: Would you say that a therapist dealing with adolescents should be or could be much more directive than a therapist dealing with adults?

Irene Josselyn: What do you mean by "directive"? With the adolescent, there are certain situations in which direct advice is very much indicated if you don't imply that he's bad simply because he doesn't follow your advice. Giving direct advice to the adolescent is often indicated because he doesn't know where else to turn, so in that sense I think that one is justified in being direct. If one is directive in terms of one's own rigid value system, then I think this is very bad for the adolescent. You can do that with the adult and he'll choose whether or not to follow the advice. An adolescent may cling to you as if you are a lifesaver; you're not giving him a chance to develop himself.

I think that it is more a matter of how much you can direct without swallowing the adolescent, how much you can direct without destroying his own individuality, his own sense of self-identity. You can disagree with an adolescent without losing him. You can have a dialogue with him in which you're honest in what you think, but you also imply that he can be honest with you, and that you respect his capacity to make a final decision.

Question: I am getting the feeling that you probably do not prescribe a very permissive attitude in the treatment of adolescents.

Irene Josselyn: No, because I think that one of the great needs of an adolescent is the security gained from a firm word that is not a paralyzingly firm word; it is neither similar to the permissive attitude of his peers nor to the rigidity of his parents. What many adolescents are really seeking are wise limits; with our being somewhat distant from the situation we are in a better position to define wise limits than their peers or most parents are. There are a lot of parents who play this role very skillfully; they don't need a therapist. I am thinking of the adolescent who faces either a rigidity or an overpermissiveness in his parents. I meet both types. Adolescents of today are very frightened by the permissiveness of some parents; they don't know what to do.

Question: There is evidence to support the impression that a growing number of adolescents are being referred for treatment and help to hospitals and clinics. Recently, there have been a large number of what I would call nonpsychiatric professionals and even some nonprofessionals who have moved into the field of helping adolescents. Do you support the provision of psychotherapy to disturbed adolescents by nonpsychiatrists, such as social workers, psychologists, and teachers, and if you do, do you see any dangers in this?

Irene Josselyn: Yes, I see dangers in psychotherapy by everyone, including psychiatrists, especially in overidentifying with the adolescent. I think that we all get caught in this. I believe that most psychiatrists have some safeguards against this, but I'm not sure about members of the other professions.

I am concerned about some psychotherapists who want to make deep dynamic interpretations to the adolescent. This can be pretty frightening to the adolescent because he is not ready to handle such problems. This approach may be more common among the nonpsychiatrists than among the psychiatrists. On the other hand, what many adolescents need most of all is a wise friend. I am probably a little more tolerant of the nonprofessional group than some of my colleagues are.

For instance, a teacher in high school who is a mature person can be an extremely significant person to an adolescent, if that mature person is willing to recognize that certain problems come up that are beyond his ability to handle and then will see the need of seeking professional help. This is ideal.

However, I would like to go back to your statement that there are more and more adolescents being referred; I am sure that today's adolescent is more overtly confused and shows it more than the adolescent of former years, but it wasn't so many years ago that a lot of the cases similar to many that we see today were evaluated as "just adolescent" and the patients were allowed to grow up. People were more tolerant really of the "diagnosis" of "adolescence" than they are now; if adolescence was the diagnosis it was assumed one didn't worry because the youth would get over it, and we'd just pretend it didn't exist.

Many adolescents being referred to us now are no different from those who formerly were not referred because they were considered "just adolescence." Although increasing our number of referrals, it's good they are being referred because I think that they can get over the hump more easily than without therapy. This is why I regard a large percentage of therapy with the adolescent as not really therapy for a pathologic condition but preventive. I look upon much of my work with adolescents really as that of preventing a crystallization in adulthood of something that is a normal part of the fluid state of adolescence.

Question: I gather that you are not opposed to nonprofessionals helping adolescents by psychotherapy or counseling. Would you try to list the dangers that nonprofessionals could run into in helping adolescents?

Irene   Well, I guess the first thing I would warn
Josselyn: them about is not to get too frightened by what the adolescent says, reacting in the

context of that fear too quickly and stepping in. It is important to listen, and to listen long enough so that what the adolescent is really saying is understood.

There is another area to consider, and I am not sure what yardstick should be used to prevent unfortunate consequences in this area. The councelors, particularly those who are nonprofessionals or who are seen as nonprofessionals by the adolescent, have to recognize the possibility of an intense emotional response on the part of the adolescent—the so-called adolescent "crush." The adult often becomes very frightened by this and pushes the adolescent off, viewing the response as sexual. It is sexual, but the sexual aspect is very secondary. If an adolescent develops a crush he is indicating that he has a great need for someone. The danger in this situation is that if the adult accepts the adolescent's need he often feels gratification and will want to swallow up the adolescent and make him into the adult's image, losing sight of the fact that he is dealing with an individual who may have a different image of the adult, and may want a different image of himself.

It has been my experience that this is really the most ticklish area encountered by nonprofessionals working with adolescents. The nonprofessionals either become frightened by the intense relationship, or they take advantage of it; they don't remain objective enough about it to help the adolescent over this pyramid.

Question: Are you saying that overidentification with the adolescent is a danger in helping adolescents?

Irene Josselyn: It is difficult for people to realize they have overidentified with a patient. All of us get patients with whom we overidentify and don't realize we have done so. This is very important to guard against because if we overidentify with an adolescent we go to their level.

This is perhaps a good time to express my definition of empathy. Empathy is a capacity to identify and then step back and look at the situation. The person who is most skillful in any therapy is the person who is able to identify and then look at what he has experienced in the identification before he acts. You can call it transference or counter-transference; I don't know what to call it, but this is what happens in a good therapeutic relationship. All of us have a nostalgia for our adolescence. We have forgotten the unpleasant things about it and we want to go back to it, which may result in the possibility of overidentification and therefore loss of our skill in empathizing, in listening and then stepping back and looking at what we have heard in terms of what the adolescent is *really* saying, not what we think he is saying.

Question: I want to bring in the term "turmoil"
because, as you know, Anna Freud (1969)
has used this term and stated that turmoil is
an essential part of growing up—I think
she went so far as to say that an adolescent
who does not show turmoil could be considered a sick adolescent. What would be
your views on this?

Irene   I don't know whether I would say that he is
Josselyn: a sick adolescent; I would rather say that
he is fixated at a preadolescent state. As I
read some of the recent literature criticizing
this attitude about adolescence it suddenly
dawned on me that there is a semantic
problem. I have been quoted as not believing
that all adolescents are in turmoil; I couldn't
understand that interpretation of my
writing until I read further. Then I realized that turmoil was being described as
a state of mental illness, of acting out, or
something that is extremely manifest. Many
of our adolescents are in turmoil, but
silently so. They are working it out while
adults are relatively unaware of what they
are working out. They are not clinging to
their childhood, they are struggling to
reach adulthood and struggling to correct
some of their childhood concepts in order
to have adult concepts; they don't show
this to us. If you happen to get to know them
as a friend rather than their having been
referred to you as a therapist, and you can
sit down to chat with them about many
things, you begin to get evidence of their
turmoil, what is going on inside of them

that is not showing in any gross manifestation.

Many of them are very healthy kids; they will reach a solution. They will listen to many people but we won't know if what they hear will help them resolve their turmoil. If you see turmoil as something pathologic then I would agree that not all adolescents go through a period of turmoil. I do think that the normal process of adolescence is a period of confusion and realignment.

Question: Would you say that adolescence is a period of unhappiness?

Irene Josselyn: It is a time of very deep unhappiness and very rich happiness. This is part of the adolescent's confusion. He feels everything so intensely. When he is unhappy he is deeply unhappy; when he is happy he is ecstatic. This is as it should be because he is feeling out things.

I have been interested for many years in my work with adults in analysis in that the picture of their adolescence that I get at the end of their analysis is often in sharp contrast to the one they have given me in their original history. They initially describe their adolescence as either all miserable or without any problems. Toward the end of the analysis they typically return to the adolescent material and then the evidence of the conflict that made them either see the period in their memory as totally unhappy or totally happy becomes clear. I have never analyzed an adult who returned to this adolescent material in whom I didn't find a different picture of his adolescence than the one he gave initially. I think that we have a repression for our own adolescence, as we have for our first five years of life.

Question: About this controversy of adolescents going through turmoil, are you suggesting that it is a matter of definition?

Irene   Yes, I think to a large extent that it's a
Josselyn: matter of definition. On the other hand, I believe that after World War II particularly, although the trend started before that, we had some generations of people, chronologically adolescent, who didn't become psychologically adolescent. As I see it, part of the present adolescent protest against materialism, or some of the other things the youths are protesting about, is a justified protest. Many of the adults never had the enriching experience of their own adolescence. They accepted the standards of their parents and the culture; they didn't wish for any change.

I can remember not so many years ago talking to some university people who expressed concern over the fact that the college students were so compliant. I imagine they now wish that they could get half of that compliancy back, but that compliance was a bad sign. Those young people apparently were geared to the idea that you obtain a college education to get a good job. You didn't have to grow up to do this; all you had to do was to get a good job. You could do that if you got a college education. I do think we went through a period in which most young people never went through adolescence. Some of the studies made at that time are used to prove that the adolescents were not mixed-up; I think they weren't mixed up because they weren't adolescents.

Question: The present adolescents are not only questioning and protesting and challenging, but they are also using drugs. How do you evaluate this phenomenon of taking drugs?

**Irene
Josselyn:**   I see it as a problem that has to be separated into its component parts; no generalization is valid.

Of the groups of drug users with whom I have had experience, there are some adolescents who use drugs primarily because adults don't think that this is a good idea. This is a subcultural phenomenon—if parents say something isn't good, then there must be something good about it; the way to grow up is to think that your parents' attitudes are wrong. The great stress on drugs by adults has tended, among a certain group of adolescents, to foster the use of drugs; that is one way of rebelling, although certainly an unfortunate way.

There is another group of adolescents who are using drugs, as many have commented, as an escape; it is just too hard to find what they want in the world, and the drugs give them a way out. This group is perhaps the one we should be most concerned about, indicative that its members are unable to cope with the real world and are finding a substitute. There are many other ways of finding a substitute. I don't think that we should just put the emphasis on the fact that these adolescents are using drugs, but rather on what their use of drugs signifies.

There is another group of drug-using adolescents whose behavior, I feel, is indicative of where we have failed them. I don't want to blame the educational system because it simply reflects the outline; but we'll pick on the educational system in order to show what I mean.

We have given our young people, through their current education, very little experience with good teachers who love the subjects that they teach and who stimulate emotional gratification from learning rather than demand factual learning only. The adolescent in his idealism and his sensitivity wants something that is beautiful. Some young people are using drugs because they don't know where else to find beauty; their background has given them mechanical learning rather than an emotional experience in learning. We certainly are not going to find an easy way to help this group. I do think that our early educational system has to be thought through again. With the demand for teachers, with the need to use many people not fully qualified as teachers, we are not getting dedicated teachers. Children are being taught facts, but not given a true educational experience. Certain adolescents are seeking in the use of drugs what they did not find through education.

I don't think that the "drug culture," as it is obten referred to in the current situation, should be called by that name. We should try to find out why a particular individual is taking drugs and what answer he is obtaining from the drug that he's not finding elsewhere. We should not be casual about the use of drugs, but I think we are overanxious. In my own experience, most of the young people I have seen over a long enough period of time have lost interest in drugs (and I don't take credit for this because of therapy, but rather attribute it to the fact they have begun to find themselves). In my opinion, at the present time, too much emphasis is being placed on how all these kids who are now using drugs are going to go on to heroin. This is creating an unnecessary panic.

Question: Are you saying that the adult society, by focusing on drugs as the issue, is almost encouraging the adolescents to use them?

Irene Josselyn: I think that is true in a certain percentage of adolescents. The adult protest is encouraging certain adolescents to use drugs because the adolescents see this as one place that they can rebel and everyone will know they are rebelling. There is no use rebelling unless people know you are rebelling, and thus this is giving them a good opportunity.

Of course there is another thing they all complain about—and in this they certainly are right. Originally when people became concerned about drugs, adults were not honest with young people. The young people were told of gruesome effects of the drugs without evidence that the stories were true. Adults have had to backtrack on a lot of what they said, so I don't blame the adolescents for being skeptical about what is said now. I have had adolescents say to me, "I heard how awful LSD was, I heard how awful shooting Speed is, but I never believed it until my friend had a bad episode." I hate to have them learn it that way, but I think that there was so much said suggesting that everybody was going to have a bad trip on LSD, that everybody was going to go psychotic on Speed. The young people knew that everybody didn't have a bad trip; everybody didn't become psychotic on Speed; therefore, they didn't believe what we said.

Question: So there was a credibility gap?

Irene   Yes, I would say there was; once the youths
Josselyn: see one of their peers having a bad trip

or going psychotic, then they look upon drugs differently.

Question: Well, in response to this drug problem a large number of approaches are being used, drop-in clinics, walk-in clinics and street work programs with youth are being developed. What do you think of these developments? The philosophy behind some of the clinics is that the young people who are alienated from the society will not seek the establishied channels of help, such as hospitals, which society has set up. Do you feel that this approach of developing special clinics, special centers, special walk-in clinics and drop-in clinics is a move in the right direction—is it the right way to cope with this problem?

Irene   The young people feel alienated and do not
Josselyn: trust the Establishment. Hospitals and out-patient clinics represent this Establishment and the young people are reluctant to go for help to these established places. In some centers in the United States, in Canada and in other countries, clinics are being set up which are being run by young medical students, young youth workers. They do not represent the Establishment.

Particularly with members of the drug group, there are situations in which the fact that they could go to talk with their peers, although slightly older than they, is productive if (and this is the big "if" that frightens me about this program) the people who are the helping persons, regardless of their' age and other factors, are really aware of the dynamite with which they are dealing and if they know what to do with it.

I know of one situation which, on the surface, seemed to represent an excellent set-up. The orientation was religious, one the young people in their desperation accepted it. Originally it seemed as if it were perhaps bringing a constructive force into this group. But then it became apparent that those who were the key people were very sick people. Religion became a neurotic solution to and underlying problem, not a constructive solution. The participants went from drug interest to a fanatic religious interest; it left the young person who sought help still very disturbed.

When psychologically healthy individuals handle these set-ups, I get the impression that very good things are being done; when the guidelines are those established by sick people, then I think there is great danger because some of the drug-using youth need real help, not just another mixed-up version of help. If the people who are active in these projects know what they are dealing with and can be careful in what they are fostering, the organizations are good; but when the work is done for some fanatic reason of the leaders, it is dangerous.

Question: In your experience, would you say that

there are some very distinct differentiating features in treating a preadolescent, for example, a 6-year-old child who is very disturbed, as compared with a 16-year-old adolescent who is very disturbed?

Irene Josselyn: Well, there is one outstanding difference as I see it and that is that the parents, except those who are very inadequate, are effective allies in the treatment of a child. The parent is the alter-ego of the child, and such a parent is one to count on, both by the child and the therapist.

With the adolescent, the person who was a strength in his childhood may be the source of the difficulty. You may find that, no matter how well-meaning the parent is, he or she is not going to be a part of the strength of the therapy. He or she may prove to be unintentionally the source of sabotage in therapy. The therapist is caught in the peculiar dilemma of dealing with an adolescent who does not have the mature strength that makes it possible to deal with him separate from his parents, or separate from his environment. At the same time the therapist doesn't have the support, the theoretical support, from the environment that he had in dealing with the younger child. The therapist is really between two horns of a dilemma, so to speak, except that the analogy is not quite adequate. With two horns there is always a space between, one doesn't have to rest on either horn, one can rest in the middle. That is adolescent therapy; one is resting in the middle. The adolescent can't be seen as an adult and he can't be seen as a child; he is halfway between.

Another aspect is that, even though I am a child analyst, I do feel that in work with children there is much that can be done in terms of parental education. Parents will modify their approach to the child without the child gaining insight into what the basic problem is. By the time the individual is caught in his adolescent mix-up, reeducating the parents will help relieve some of the strain, but I question whether all the strain can be relieved. The adolescent himself needs help.

Another aspect is that in adolescent therapy where you are being effective and the adolescent accepts it, you become more emotionally meaningful to the adolescent than you do to the child. In child therapy you may be very meaningful to the child but you never replace the parents, if the parents have anything positive to offer. In working with adolescents, you often get a relationship with your patient in which, and this is one of the danger points in which you have to be very skillful, you do not become the parent but as emotionally meaningful to the adolescent as the parent used to be. This not only gives you an additional tool but it also gives you a dangerous tool if you don't know how to handle it.

Question: Another dilemma that I see in terms of treatment of adolescents is that, although you are treating the adolescent (and here I am really talking about treating the adolescent in private practice), in most cases the bill is being paid by the parents. Do you feel that the fact that you are paid by the father, whom the adolescent hates, creates any problems in therapy?

Irene Josselyn: I think that adolescents use this fact but I'm not sure that it is a valid use. I'm not sure that the fact that the parent pays is really the problem. The adolescent may say, "The only reason you are seeing me is because my Dad pays for it." This may tempt the therapist to say, "Well, I'll see you for nothing." This would not solve anything because what is really being expressed is some uneasiness, either anger at the therapist or the result of feeling too tied to the therapist. The adolescent has to do something to dilute the relationship, by either being angry or depreciating the personal value of the therapist. He loves to trick the therapist with this.

I had an adolescent who came for therapy very conscientiously and always kept telling me what a waste of time it was. I asked him one day why he kept coming if it was such a waste of time. He answered that it was because his father griped everytime he got my bill. My immediate reaction was to be defensive. Then I realized that this boy was saying something; he couldn't tell me that he wanted to keep coming unless he could give some negative reason for coming. After all he could have found other ways to cost his father money, he didn't have to have my bill. We finally got the situation worked out.

You see here, perhaps, the analyst's philosophy is chiefly to blame. There is always the statement that unless the patient pays, and it hurts a little bit to pay for his therapy, it isn't going to do any good. I've often wondered under those circumstances why a psychiatrist ever treats a millionaire. It doesn't hurt a millionaire to pay a medical bill—most of it is deducted from his income tax. He pays less for his therapy than a patient does who pays a full fee or even pays a half fee and has an income of $7,000 a year. I have never known of anyone who refused to treat a patient because he was a millionaire. We can get trapped into this paying business. Sometimes parents will gripe about the bill and say that therapy is not doing any good. So why does their child keep going if it is not doing any good? But the parents don't stop the therapy. I have had many adolescents report such a conversation with their parents saying that they didn't know what to do. We should look back behind the idea about parents not paying as a factor in therapy.

Question: Do you feel there is a value in follow-up of the adolescents whom one has treated?

**Irene
Josselyn:**

It is extremely worthwhile. If one can get through the day-by-day anxieties and have a little perspective, adolescents are perhaps the most rewarding age group to deal with; you don't realize that until 10 years later. You don't realize it at the time because it seems like the hardest type of therapy. I also feel very strongly that we should consider adolescence as a phase that most people will survive. Many of the adolescents of today whom we are deeply concerned about are going to be good, constructive adults.

With our awareness now of the multiple problems that the adolescent faces we are in real danger of being pessimistic about them; I don't think this is warranted. Adolescents are going to struggle through their adolescence, and a large percentage of them are going to reach maturity, and as a result of that they will make the world better than the one they entered, just as I hope that we improved the world we entered. There is a progressive phenomenon in our culture manifested through the years that, in my opinion, can be attributed to the growth that occurs in adolescence. It is the adolescent who defines new ideals; he can put them into practice on a realistic basis in adulthood. As he expresses his ideals in adolescence he is naive, inexperienced and unrealistic, but when he matures his ideals become wisdom.

The greatest danger for the adolescent today

is that in our attempt to bring some sense into our present chaos, we are going to be unwisely repressive. Repression of the adolescent will damage the future, just as repression has prevented the growth of primitive cultures in which the adolescent must follow rigidly the mores of his forebears.

REFERENCE

Freud, Anna (1969): Adolescence as a Developmental Disturbance. In: *Psychosocial Perspectives,* G. Caplan and S. Lebovici, Eds. Basic Books, Inc., New York.

Chapter 6

PSYCHOSIS AND SEVERE
NEUROSIS IN YOUTH

William M. Easson

When an adolescent is labeled psychotic or severely
neurotic, there is usually a great deal of pressure to
"treat" him, to change his behavior in some way, to do
something with him—at times almost to do anything. Since
this pressure comes from the community, from the teenager's family and sometimes even from the adolescent
himself, the helping professional may feel that he has
to act quickly and decisively. The judge and the lawyer
want to be told what is best for this teenager. The school
principal and the teachers do not know whether he should
be in school and want someone to instruct them. People
say he should be in jail and the sheriff asks what can be
done with him. The parents cannot control her—tolerate
him—understand them—and need help. The professional
must be very cautious before he makes diagnostic statements or prescribes treatment. He should know exactly
what he is doing, why he is taking this course of action
that people call "treatment" and what will be the result
of this treatment.

In the teenager's life there are definite reasons why he is neurotic or psychotic. Though his behavior is now called "sick," this sick way of life has been useful to him. In some way his neurosis, his psychosis, has helped this teenager cope with the special stresses of his life; this way of living has been rewarding or relieving in some fashion; this individual life style has developed in response to the behavior and the expectations of the people around him. Before there is any action, any treatment, it is necessary first to discover how the youth's pattern of living—which is now unacceptable in some way—has allowed him to exist and to be what he wants to be, and what pleasure, relief or reward this life style has brought. The members of the caring-treatment team must clarify who is disturbed by the youth's behavior. They must find out what it is precisely that he does, thinks or appears to be that makes people anxious or angry. Before the neurotic or psychotic teenager is expected or required to change the way he lives, it is necessary to know what effect such change may bring and whether the teenager can indeed change. Can he change his way of living very much and still remain the kind of person he himself likes? Can he change his behavior and still continue to be a member of his own family? Can he change and still be accepted by his peer group and his community?

THE EVALUATION

The adolescent's ability to cope emotionally and to grow has depended all along on:

1. The strength of his personality, his self-confidence, his ego strength.

2. The stress and the responsibilities placed on him by his own inner needs and drives, by the expectations of those around him, and by the demands of his community and culture.

3. The patterns and the style of behavior that he has "learned" during his developmental years.

4. His ability to use external support and direction, his relationship ability.

In the development of the youth's personality, these four factors are closely interdependent and overlapping. Before any definitive management or treatment decisions are made, the professional must have a clear concept of how the adolescent's growth has been encouraged, stunted or distorted by these factors in his development, factors that may very well be continuing. In order to get this information and to clarify these issues, the evaluating team must use every source of information available to it.

Communication by the Teenager

Most normal adolescents hesitate to talk openly about their uncertainties and anxieties. They feel, with good reason, that their private feelings are their private concerns. At this stage in their growth, they do not wish to appear vulnerable or inadequate. They want to test out their emotions and their ideas further before they have to share them. If a teenager *can* discuss his inner strivings and deeper emotions, he is either very healthy or very sick. When an adolescent talks very openly about his fears and his hopes, the interviewer must ask himself whether this young man has so much self-confidence, such excellent self-control, that he has no need of further evaluation or treatment; on the other hand, the interviewer must question whether this very open and verbal adolescent has so little emotional strength and such limited self-control that he cannot hold back his private feelings and thus must be very sick indeed.

Certain cultural groups in our society normally communicate more through nonverbal language. For instance, members of the Jewish or Italian communities speak more in their hand gestures and their facial expression than in words. The Negro uses body language and the language of dress when he shares his feelings and ideas. Usually the young person who is emotionally ill or disturbed is limited in his ability to communicate through words. While most teenage patients just cannot talk and will not talk, yet they will share themselves in many other forms of interaction. This adolescent, who is said to be disturbed, is now being evaluated because his communication in the past has been blocked, distorted or misunderstood—due either to the way he communicates or to the inability of those around him to understand exactly what he is communicating. The evaluating professional team should be able to use a wide range of nonverbal communications in their evaluation process, but, at the same time, they must be very clear as to what exactly is being communicated and when there is communication. The interviewer must be able to hear, to see and to feel what the teenager is trying to tell about himself.

Though the adolescent may say a great deal in words—words exploding out, words filled with love or hate, words that ring with the slogans of his culture and his time—that teenager may reveal even more in the quality and the tone of these words. Often it is very useful to listen not to the actual words that the teenager is mouthing but rather to the sound of these words. When the adolescent is talking about his mother in a dull monotone, though he is using many emotionally loaded words about this relationship, the listener must ask himself why these words are monotonous—where is the real feeling, the love and the hate—is there feeling—should there be any emotions in this situation? When the adolescent talks about something he calls "loneliness," he may use many words, he may use very few words, but the interviewer must try to sense from these words—and the gestures and the expressions the teenager uses as he talks—whether this is loneliness of good things that are now past, or whether this is the loneliness of things that never have been. When the teenager describes himself as "depressed," the evaluating team must know what this word really feels to him. Is this a depression about people and experiences that have gone and are now no more or is this the depression of inadequacy, inability and being overwhelmed? When the young teenager speaks about being "happy," what is the quality of this word? What is this emotion he calls happiness? Is this the happiness that comes when other people leave him alone, is this the kind of happiness that is merely the relief of sadness and of pain, or is this the happiness of caring for others and being cared for by them? When the adolescent mentions that he has been "confused," the interviewer must ask himself who taught the teenager this word and what does it mean to him. Is this his confusion or is this the confusion of the people around him? Was he right when they were wrong—or were they all wrong—or were they right and wrong—and confused?

The words and the phrases of the disturbed teenager may say a great deal or may say very little, but usually he tells much more about himself in the way he looks, in the gestures of his hands, in the expression of his face and in the posture of his body. His words may be bland and reassuring, but his uneasy movements as he sits there in his chair may speak more eloquently about the anxiety and the anguish he feels. He may talk about the misery he has lived through and seem to be self-confident, yet the way he sits so rigidly in his chair may indicate how tightly he has had to keep his inner anxiety under control—and the dark, lonely anguish of his eyes and the slight quiver of his mouth may show how close this anxiety is to awareness and how fragile is his rigid control. The adolescent may tell the interviewer that he is happy—gloriously happy—deliriously happy—and he may smile comfortably and his clothes may be bright and colorful and then the interviewer will be able to believe this happiness, but sometimes a teenager will talk about happiness and pleasure and his clothes are dismal and drab and give another message, a message of sadness and despair, a more meaningful message. The young adolescent may emphasize repeatedly that his life is organized and planned and the words he uses may be precise and appropriate, but his hair may be awry and his clothing disorganized and disheveled; the interviewer should know then that this adolescent may be really rather disorganized inside—because the teenager will have communicated this message nonverbally and the helping professional should be able to understand what is being told.

Communication from Others

The teenager may pull himself together emotionally and be the picture of charm, organization and self-sufficiency for any interview or series of interviews. He may keep up this appearance of maturity for quite some time. Very often the members of the interviewing team are so impressed by the way the adolescent appears in one or two short sessions that they do not allow themselves to appreciate the communications they are receiving about the adolescent's way of life outside these interviews. Because the caring professional wishes to help this adolescent, he may need to see the teenager as more ready to be helped than he really is. Since the professional, as a caring human being, wants to care, he may allow himself to think that this adolescent is ready and willing to accept his care. What appears to be the teenager's self-confidence and self-assertiveness in the interview may be merely the adolescent's ability to pick up the cues that are readily and sometimes eagerly provided by the evaluation team members. The teenager may have become an excellent manipulator through years of experience, and what seems to be the adolescent's warmth and enthusiasm in the interviews may only be his manipulative charm. The youngster's anger seen during the interview may not be rage aroused by a specific topic or interviewer, but rather may be a primitive defense against anxiety aroused in any interaction. To understand the interviews more completely, the evaluation team must use a wide range of communications from outside these interview sessions to confirm and to explain the communications seen, felt and heard during the sessions with the adolescent.

It is essential that the evaluating team gets as extensive a history as possible of the teenager's development and of the way he functions out there in society. No definitive final treatment decisions should be made—no matter what pressures there are—until there is a clear history. The youth professional must know what the teenager's parents have to say about his development and about his present way of life. He must know how the adolescent did in school, whether he had a job and what happened to him on the job. He must know what his school grades were and why. He must know what the teenager does with himself and with other people. How much individuality does the adolescent show and what response does he get? How do people react to him and what does he do when they do react?

Sometimes the interviewer feels that, in order to be an acceptable ally to the adolescent, he has to disregard the statements and the opinions of other people. The professional may justify this attitude by saying that other people in some way are biased against the adolescent. Certainly this background information will be biased, but the teenager's communications are also biased and the biases of all these people are in part a product of the teenager's behavior in the past and his present personality.

The interviewer must allow himself to receive, to understand and to integrate all communications about this adolescent who is said to be disturbed. The evaluating team should seek reports from schools, from doctors, from employers, from ministers. They should listen to neighbors, uncles, aunts and grandparents—to anyone who has known or who has been affected by this adolescent. These communications from other people will tell how this teenager has developed and how he has been able to function in his society. He comes to the evaluating team, a product of his developmental years, and the evaluating team must know what happened during those years of growth because that knowledge will tell them where the adolescent is emotionally and what he might be able to do.

Communication from the Interviewer Himself

The interviewer and the adolescent have the opportunity to feel exactly what effect the adolescent has on other people in the interview sessions. The interviewer must permit himself to experience and to use this form of direct communication. He has to allow himself to respond to the teenager and then evaluate his own reactions so that he can gauge the effect of this adolescent on the people around him. The interview is a small sample of how this adolescent functions and how he interacts. As one interacting human being, the interviewer can use himself as a clinical example of what the teenager does to people.

The professional must ask himself whether he finds that he is drawing closer emotionally to the adolescent as he and the youth talk together or whether he feels that he is being pushed away and closed out. Does he find that he is receiving a confusing message—is he being drawn closer and pushed away at the same time? Is he having conflicting feelings about this teenager? What are these communications that he feels he is getting from the adolescent? What messages is he responding to as he talks to this young person? When he is with this teenager does the interviewer feel empathic, anxious, angry or bored—and why? As the interviews progress, does the professional find himself restless and uneasy—and what then is happening between him and the teenager? Does this adolescent have the emotional ability to make people want to give to him and does the interviewer feel this appeal working on himself? How does the teenager relate—aggressively, passively, intrusively—and is this way of relating attractive or repellent to another human being? What is the quality of this teenager's sexuality? How does the interviewer find himself responding to this adolescent as a young man or as a young woman?

When he is with this disturbed adolescent, the caring-evaluating professional should be able to sense the effect of this teenager on the people around him. If this adolescent is indeed neurotic or psychotic, this maladaptive pattern of behavior should be shown in the way he interacts with those around him—and thus in the effect that he has on the interviewer in the interview setting. So often people who are neurotic or psychotic make others uneasy or uncomfortable and eventually are rejected by those people who say they care. The interviewer should be able to sense whether he also is tempted to push the adolescent away and to reject him even while he is saying that he wants to understand and to help, and he should question what factors lead to this reaction.

The adolescent will also tend to deal with the interviewer in the same way the teenager has been treated by meaningful people in his life. The professional person may find that, during the interviews, he is beginning to experience the kind of life situation the teenager lives through constantly in his world outside. If this adolescent is given constantly confusing messages he will also tend to spread confusion and distortion and thus, during the evaluation, the youth professional may begin to sense that somehow he also is becoming confused. If the disturbed adolescent constantly receives threatening, anxiety-provoking communications from the people around him, he will also arouse anxiety in the way he interacts with other people—and he will spread this anxiety to the examiner in the examination process. In this limited way, the interviewing team members may be able to experience with the teenager some of the emotional realities he has to live through in the world outside the examining treatment sessions.

The evaluating team should then put together the communications that they have received from the adolescent, from the people who interact with the adolescent and from their own interactions with the teenager; these communications should tell what kind of person this disturbed adolescent is or should highlight questions that have yet to be answered. The evaluation process should allow the professional team to understand the meaning of the teenager's behavior and, on the basis of this understanding, to suggest how this disturbed adolescent and his community can be helped best.

In dealing with the severely disturbed adolescent, it is helpful to consider the emotional disturbances of adolescence in different categories even though these overlap widely.

THE ADOLESCENT WITH INADEQUATE PERSONALITY STRENGTH

The adolescent who is disturbed and disturbing because he does not have the emotional strength to deal with the stresses of his day-to-day living may present a wide range of neurotic or psychotic symptoms. This symptom picture, due to personality inadequacy, may arise in the adolescent who has normal emotional strengths but faces overwhelming stress or in the adolescent who is facing normal stresses of the teenage years with stunted, limited and underdeveloped personality capabilities.

The emotional growth of the adolescent may have been normal, but the stress he now faces is beyond the normal capacity of the average adolescent. The emotional burden he faces is excessive and would overwhelm any other teenager with normal emotional capabilities. The teenager's normal emotional strength is thus relatively inadequate to deal with excessive stress. On the other hand, there are many teenagers whose emotional strength is so limited that they cannot cope with even normal life stresses. In face of the routine expectations and responsibilities of the adolescent years, these teenagers are unable to function adequately.

From the information given by the teenager, from the way he presents himself and from his developmental history, it should be possible to ascertain which type of personality inadequacy this adolescent is now manifesting.

The Adolescent with Inadequate Personality Strength Dealing with Normal Life Stresses

During his developmental years, the teenager may have found it difficult or even impossible to develop reasonable, stable ways of reacting to the people and to the happenings around him. In his childhood he may have been faced with too many anxieties and too much confusion to allow him to develop firm opinions and adequate self-confidence. During these growth years when he tried to be independent and attempted to express his individuality, he may have met with repeated rejection and anger from the caring people in his life. His parents and his family may have been unable or unwilling to give him consistent direction and control. By adolescence his emotional development will then have been uneven, uncertain and stunted; he will be less able to tolerate the normal stresses of the teenage years and to use the upsurge of adolescent energy for growth.

There are certain children who are more prone than others to develop an unstable inadequate personality. The child who has been overdependent on another stronger, controlling person during his childhood years may be unable to function adequately as an independent adolescent. If a child has continued to be very close to mother or to father, this closeness may have been maintained at the cost of the child's own emotional self-sufficiency. Mother's boy may have stayed so close to mother emotionally that the young man finds that he has never really developed his own opinions and ideas. The cute little girl may have been so charming and lovable and so protected by her family that she never had to learn on her own and, because she never had to learn, she never developed the ability to cope with ordinary life stresses. When a parent and a child have clung to each other emotionally, this clinging relationship may have been emotionally rewarding to both during the years of childhood, but this closeness may have prevented the child—and indeed the parent also —from developing the necessary self-confidence and self-sufficiency necessary to be independent in adolescence.

A 17-year-old young man asked to see a psychiatrist because "he did not know what to do." This boy, now in his senior year of high school, somehow found himself unable to make decisions. He described himself as "powerless." He was constantly restless and vaguely depressed. He found it more and more difficult to "gather his thoughts."

This teenager was the only son and younger child of two socially active professional parents. The family came from a minority ethnic group and, though they were very successful socially and financially, they tended to keep to themselves. In their very comfortable home environment this adolescent and his parents "shared everything"— they knew about each other's hopes and fears, anxieties and strivings. No matter what this boy did he always consulted his parents. This was a very warm and gratifying family relationship for the parents and their son.

Though these parents encouraged him "to do things on his own," they still continued to plan with him just what he should do. One week before this consultation, this young man had invited his girlfriend over to his home for the evening. His parents deliberately went out for those hours. His mother had made sure that a very nice meal was laid out and that a bottle of wine was provided. Just that afternoon his father had asked his son whether the teenager was planning to have sexual intercourse with his girlfriend that evening; the father gently suggested that the young man should provide himself with contraceptives. Though the young man had some vague idea that something sexual might occur during the evening, he had had no previous heterosexual experience. After this discussion with his father, he did go out and buy contraceptives.

That evening, after a very successful meal and a very relaxed, happy discussion, the young man and his girlfriend went to bed together—in the parental bedroom—and there, strange to relate, the young man found that he was impotent. He worried about his impotence for the next week and he wondered what it all meant in terms of his "virility." He could not sleep at night. He could not do his school work. He was crying "without apparent reason." Suicidal thoughts began to drift into his mind. He feared that he "might do something to himself." He felt that he was "going to explode." Without consulting his parents he sought psychiatric help.

In reality this adolescent was psychologically impotent as well as physically impotent. Because he and his parents had had such a close relationship, he had never been allowed nor had he allowed himself to develop his own independent opinions and his own self-confidence. When suddenly reality faced him with the fact that he was not self-sufficient, his anxieties began to mount and as the tension mounted he was less and less able to cope. He began to show increasing neurotic symptoms. Even in this very "good" family, this teenager had grown up without the normal personality strength of the average adolescent. In a normally stressful situation, he was unable to cope.

There are many reasons why parents tend to hold on

to their children emotionally and why children cling to their parents. Often a youngster is felt to be special or precious in some way. There is good cause why he should be protected and shielded. He may be the youngest, the oldest, the first or the last. He may be the only boy, she may be the only girl. Other children may have died. He may have had an illness that threatened his life. She may be asthmatic. He may have a heart complaint or a physical deformity. The parents may be lonely, alone and unappreciated by the people around them. Mother may need someone to love her and her little girl may give her that love. Father may feel unsuccessful in his job but knows that his young son always admires him. The parents may be bored with each other but find that their youngster is always understanding and enthusiastic. During the child's developmental years, this close relationship with a parent —or indeed a close relationship with any other person— may have been mutually enriching to the child and to the other person, but this enrichment may come at the expense of the child's own self-sufficiency. Because the growing child is so very close, he may never develop the kind of self-confidence and self-control that he needs in order to become an independent adequate adolescent. During the teenage years he—or she—may then be unable to cope independently and may "present" with a neurosis or even with a psychotic reaction in face of the normal stresses of the teenage years.

Some children seem to be constitutionally more liable to lack the confidence and self-control necessary to cope with adolescent stresses than others. Certain children seem to be born with unusually strong drives or instinctual needs. They may demand more than their parents—even normal parents—can give. They may need more control and guidance than the parents can provide. There are parents who enjoy having a youngster who is infantile and therefore these parents encourage childish behavior.

But when their child becomes an adolescent, his aggressive, demanding child-like behavior may be too much for the family or for the teenager's community to tolerate. He may then be told quite suddenly to control his behavior and to conform to the standards of those around him. He is now given responsibilities and he is expected to cope. With only the emotional strength and the self-control of a very young child, this infantile teenager is now required to function as a self-sufficient young man or young woman. These age-appropriate expectations are beyond his emotional capabilities. He cannot grow up all at once. His anxiety begins to spiral. He cannot manage. He begins to show increasingly disturbed behavior. He may decompensate emotionally in explosive neurotic or psychotic reactions.

When he was a child, John "ran wild" on his family ranch. During his grade-school years, he "just got by" in school. He was able to contain himself long enough in the classroom to get through his classes and then he would be outside "fighting and storming and doing." His family enjoyed his constant "boyish" activity and gave him the full freedom of the ranch.

But when he became a teenager, John began to run into difficulties. His parents found that his threats and his demands were no longer cute—he was over 6 feet tall and he was quite capable of "giving someone a pounding." When he had a temper tantrum, this bearded muscular young man looked very ridiculous and very menacing. His classmates in school were afraid of him now and with good reason; in one angry outburst, John kicked a "friend" so hard that he broke the friend's leg. Because his peers were afraid of him, John was shunned more and more; he was even shunned by his brothers and sisters. In his loneliness he became increasingly unreasonable and depressed until one day, when he was out on the hills shooting at squirrels, he impulsively turned his gun on himself. Fortunately his hand shook at the last moment so that he only blasted off a corner of his right ear. He had not killed himself that time, but he was horribly, desperately lonely. He did not know what to do. He had no friends. He was suicidally depressed. His parents brought him for an evaluation.

The syndrome of childhood autism has been well recognized since Kanner's description in 1943. If the infant has only minimal ability to relate, if he has little "sending ability," or if his innate relationship capability is stunted very early in his growth owing to the emotional rejection of those around him, this child is liable to grow up autistic, in an emotional world of his own. By adolescence, he will be severely retarded socially and intellectually. When the autism is less absolute, this youngster may, in the adolescent years, present a pervasive neurosis or a schizophrenia.

This autistic syndrome is well recognized, but there is a comparable behavior pattern that is much more frequent and can be equally disabling. The child who grows up with "excessive sending power" may be just as handicapped as the autistic child who has minimal ability to relate. The growing youngster, with excessive sending power, has the ability to charm other people into doing things for him. He is so cute that others "just love" to care for him, to protect him and to tell him what to do, so that he is very liable to grow up without ever learning how to do the most simple, most basic things on his own. If the child continues to be so charming as he grows that the people around him protect him all the time, he will have little opportunity and need to develop his own emotional strength and his own independence. He will continue to be cute and charming because he will learn very early that this attractiveness makes other people very happy and brings him many rewards.

With the onset of adolescence, such a child may no longer appear quite as charming to the people around him.

His attractiveness may take on a quality that is now disturbing. The cuteness may be more sexual or more aggressive and thus more frightening. The family members, the neighbors, the teachers who used to be charmed may become more distant. In the teenage years the youngster who was so cute may find that he has to start making his own decisions and planning his own life—without ever having had this kind of experience before. Until this time the schoolteachers have tended to give him the easier questions because he was so charming, but now he faces the same tasks as the other adolescents and he may not be able to manage. When he was younger, the other children in the neighborhood and in his class did things for him because he was so nice, but now that he has become an adolescent they wait for him to do his share. Because he was able to charm others to decide for him, to give him directions and to do things for him, he may find that he does not know what to do when he becomes an adolescent.

The classic example of the young person who is crippled by excessive sending power is the "dumb blonde" —the young lady who has been so beautiful and so attractive that the people around her have automatically done things for her. The dumb blonde is expected only to be beautiful and, because she is beautiful, other people will open doors to her, help her to her chair and give her flowers and candy—for those are the things that you do for a dumb blonde. She is not expected to have ideas or feelings of her own and, indeed, if she does have an opinion, people will tend to look at her in wonder and dismay. She will be told that she is pretty, she is charming, and therefore it is not necessary for her to have opinions.

There are many charming teenagers who because of their charm have been able to get other people to do things for them. They have not had to develop their own personality strengths. Then, in the face of normal adolescent stresses, these teenagers who are blessed and cursed with excessive sending power may find that they just cannot cope. Their tension mounts. They begin to show pervasive neurotic symptoms. They may be unable to function. They may show psychotic decompensation.

Miklos was a charming 19-year-old. He would sit in the waiting room, smiling coyly to himself, and the secretaries would walk down the hallway just to pass by him. The receptionist noted that he read all the "hot rod" magazines so she bought new ones which she placed in the waiting room prior to his visits.

In his interviews, Miklos would look appealingly, charmingly, at the interviewer who would somehow find himself providing answers and giving cues. Miklos was attractive but was unable to function independently out there in the big wide world. He never had to ask for a car. His parents saved for several years to buy him one. They wanted to give him a car. He never had to look for girl-friends. The girls came looking for him. Even though he was rather short for his age, he was on the school basketball team "because people liked him." Yet somehow things were "beginning to go wrong." Miklos was finding that he could attract people, he could charm them, but he could not keep their friendship. He had many acquaintances but he had no friends. Plaintively he complained that "nobody knew him," but in reality there was little to know about this 19-year-old and Miklos tended to keep people from knowing how little there really was.

Everyone around him was "doing his thing" and Miklos did not have a thing to do. His classmates were becoming engaged and drifting away from him, they were going off to their jobs, to their games, to their friends— and leaving him. Even his parents did not seem to be quite as interested in him now. Just this summer they had gone off on a holiday and left him at home alone for the first time. In college he found he was becoming increasingly compulsive. Each hour he had to go back to his locker to make sure that his shoes were arranged correctly and that his jacket was hanging straight. He rearranged his locker at least three times each day and, just the previous week, he went back one evening to rearrange his locker again. He was becoming disturbed with his own feelings because he was angry at people—nasty, vicious—and "this is not like me." He had a vague general sense of sadness, of pervasive hopelessness, of "being useless."

Some children grow up and develop their opinions and their ideas merely by reacting against the opinions and the ideas of the people around them. In some youngsters this reacting-against seems to be a perpetuation of the negativism of the very young child who refuses in order to show that he has a mind of his own—the 2-year-old who says "No" when offered a cookie just to demonstrate that he can make a decision. Other children may need to react against the opinion of the people around them because emotionally they are unable or unwilling to develop their own ideas or attitudes. From all the information he receives about the adolescent, the evaluating professional must clarify as far as possible just how much the teenager's behavior is merely a response to other people and to what extent the adolescent does make up his mind and express his own ideas. Did the teenager let his hair grow long because he thought he looked attractive with long hair or did he let it grow because his father wanted him to have his hair cut short? Did he decide not to go to school just to show that he was not going to be pushed around by those teachers or did he think he would learn more in that job he has taken? Does the teenage girl wear that short skirt because it suits her and she looks attractive in it or does she wear it because her mother does not like short skirts? Are the boy and girl "in love" with each other because their parents think that they have a bad influence on each other or are they in love because they care deeply and meaningfully for one another? So often the teenager seems to be making independent meaningful decisions when, in reality, he is only opposing a decision that someone else has made. This reacting-against behavior always occurs as one part of normal teenage rebellion, but reacting-against can become so pervasive and so absolute that a teenager gets to the position of never making a decision on his own. He only reacts-against someone else's decisions and attitudes and thus he never does develop his own ideas and his own self-confidence. If he goes through adolescence merely reacting-against other people, he always needs other people to react-against in order to function. Those people, out there, always have to make the decision first and then he reacts-against their decision. When other people do not make decisions, he may have to force them to commit themselves and he often forces this commitment by being disturbing, aggressive or anxiety-provoking. The reacting-against adolescent must have other people take a stand first so that he knows what to do—by going opposite to them. If the adolescent continues in this pattern of reacting-against other people, he will develop only a pseudo-identity for himself, an identity that is totally dependent on the decisions of others, an identity that is liable to crumble when he has to face decisions that he cannot avoid.

Some adolescents grow up merely mirroring a group identity. When they were younger, they functioned as part of a family or a family group and emotionally they were carried along. In the adolescent years they attach themselves to a gang, to a crowd, to a social group, and they take the opinions, the plans and the goals of this group. When "they" think a certain style is cool, this adolescent must have this style in order to exist. When his group believes in a certain cause, he will believe in that cause without question. When a teenage girl's crowd hates a teacher, she will slavishly hate that same person—because she can only mirror the identity of her group. When this kind of teenager is separated from his or her group, family, or crowd, it may become obvious that the youth has very little self-confidence and very little inherent ability. When expected to make an independent decision, he will be unable to commit himself without the direction and the support of his group. In a desperate, frantic fashion, he may try to form a new group around him by taking a job, by going into the armed services, or even by marrying; in marriage, this kind of teenager may set up a small private group with the marriage partner making the decisions, setting the style and giving the strength—and thus giving him an identity, a borrowed personality.

When an adolescent with limited, stunted or distorted personality strength is expected to be emotionally independent and face the normal responsibilities of the teenage years, he may be unable to cope. His anxieties will mount. He may be depressed, phobic, compulsive, or develop a wide range of hysterical symptoms. He may act-out explosively. He may withdraw hopelessly. If the stress continues, even these normal stresses of the adolescent years, his inner anxiety may become so intolerable that he disintegrates emotionally and presents a psychotic syndrome.

The Adolescent with Normal Personality Development, Decompensating under Excessive Stress

There are certain life situations that may be overwhelming even for the normal healthy person—war, that overwhelming social psychosis—the unexpected, searing fire disaster—the unbearable agony that comes with the loss of the most meaningful loved one. Even a normal adolescent, who has grown up with adequate self-confidence, with a reasonable individuality and with an ability to relate comfortably to other people, even he may be faced with responsibilities and stresses that he cannot manage. In situations where the emotional demands are too great, a normal adolescent may become overwhelmingly anxious. When his anxiety starts to develop, his ability to cope effectively decreases and his anxiety then mounts even faster.

In a situation of gross, continued, unmanageable stress, where there is no escape and no apparent end in sight, a normal teenager, like any normal adult, may eventually be unable to cope. As his tension rises, he will usually first show a wide range of neurotic symptoms before he gives way to panic, to psychotic withdrawal, or to open emotional disorganization. If the stress is excessive and if there are absolutely no ways of lessening the tension by action, even a normal person may decompensate very rapidly and may quite suddenly disrupt in a profound psychotic reaction.

SYMPTOMS OF PERSONALITY INADEQUACY, RELATIVE OR ABSOLUTE

The caring professional will have to learn from all the personal history available to him whether he is dealing with a teenager who is basically inadequate and who has decompensated under normal life stresses or whether his task is to help a relatively normal, "healthy" adolescent who has been unable to deal with excessive, intolerable responsibility. These syndromes of personality inadequacy, relative and absolute, overlap and the symptoms manifested will be very similar. For meaningful treatment, it is essential to clarify what factors are operating and what strengths the adolescent has available to deal with his situation.

If the adolescent is experiencing personality inadequacy, relative or absolute, his first symptoms may well be a kind of formless, nameless anxiety—an anxiety without a focus, a vague general feeling that is "just there." Quickly, however, this anxiety may become focused on some life situation or on a person in the teenager's life—in a phobia, in compulsively driven behavior or in paranoid suspicion. In face of this rising inner anxiety, the adolescent will feel inescapably inadequate and intolerably hopeless. His tension may be directed inward; he may show depression and numbing apathy. In an attempt to deal with his mounting uncertainty, the adolescent often overreacts—he may bluster, he may challenge, he may take on even greater responsibilities. If this anxiety due to personality inadequacy continues or becomes worse, the teenager may become more and more disruptive and impulsive or he may withdraw from his peers and his family. To an increasing extent his behavior is dictated by his inner drives and his own private perceptions and ideas. Under continuing stress, the adolescent with inadequate personality—inadequate due to basic developmental defects or inadequate to cope with intolerable stress—may come for evaluation or treatment with a wide range of neurotic or psychotic symptoms.

This picture of the severely disturbed adolescent, the teenager with multiple neurotic traits or with a psychosis, is often seen in the "double-bind" situation, in that life situation where the adolescent is faced with a problem from which there is no escape, in which no matter what he does is wrong and whatever he decides will cause him to experience pain. He cannot avoid the problem. He cannot act in any way that will give him relief. When the adolescent has grown up in the family in which double-bind situations occur frequently, his own personality structure will at least in part have been formed by these repeated double binds. As he tries to deal with the impossible, unavoidable pain he faces in his family relationships, he can never escape totally because he has modeled his own behavior and his own attitudes after those of his family. He carries his own double bind with him. In order to escape an impossible situation, not only does he have to escape his own family but also he has to deny a basic part of his own personality. Thus a teenager who constantly faces double-bind family situations is likely to decompensate emotionally and to present a picture of a reactive psychosis.

> " . . . and she said to me 'Do you want a knuckle sandwich?'
>
> "I saw her teeth and she was smiling. And I wanted to go up to my room, but I knew she would come up after me. And she stood there smiling at me, her teeth—and she held her fist up like this. And then something happened to me. . . . ."

In this way a 15-year-old girl told how her psychosis began. As she said these words, she was giggling and theatrical, but she was watching suspiciously everything around her. She could not sit in her chair; she had to be up looking around to make sure that "nothing would happen." She said that she was friendly with everyone, but she had to touch all the people who came into the room, just to make sure that they were "safe." This situation she described was one of the many double-bind episodes she had lived through. This time again her own mother had placed her in a position that was intolerable, but an intolerable position from which she could not escape. So this 15-year-old girl escaped at last in the only way left open to her. She became psychotic.

Even a healthy, mature teenager will be unable to cope with some of the double-bind situations of life. These impossible, intolerable conflicts may occur in school, at the job, at home—as well as at the battle front, during that crucial examination and in face of those impossible demands made by "friends."

From all the information available to them the professional team should be able to say whether the maladaptive behavior shown by the adolescent is due to inadequate personality development, to overwhelming, intolerable stress or, as often happens, to a combination of both factors as is manifest in the double-bind interaction.

THE DISTURBED ADOLESCENT IN THE DISTURBED FAMILY

As a child is growing up he is learning his behavior from his parents, from his family and from those around him. He looks to these people for guidance and example. Over the years he finds that certain behavior is routinely rewarded in his family while other behavior brings pain or punishment. By adolescence, the youth's way of life reflects to a great extent what he has been taught over the years by his family.

In a family in which neurotic behavior is the usual style of life, the children in that family will grow up neurotic. To be nonneurotic, to be a "healthy" youngster, would mean that this child was different from his family; he would not be similar to them in the way that he behaved. Neurotic parents would be uncomfortable with a nonneurotic child.

In a phobic family whose members are taught to fear, the children grow up fearful. If the mother fears dark hallways and shadowy closets, her sons and daughters will fear darkness and shadows—even in adolescence. If the parents are scared of thunder, their children will fear thunder and their children will teach their grandchildren to fear also. The more things the parents fear, the more their child will be phobic in the teenage years. In a family in which everything is obsessively planned and regimented, the growing young boy will have this kind of obsessiveness solidly built into his character. As he has grown up, his neatness, his predictability, his firm self-control will have been repeatedly rewarded and if he tried to act more flexibly or with less predictability he would have been punished. In the paranoid family in which the parents believe that "they are against us"—whether "they" are the Communists, the Negroes, the Jews, the non-Jews or whomever mother or father feels is threatening or menacing—the teenagers in that family will also be paranoid. The young boy will have been trained through the years to be overly sensitive and suspicious; his attitudes will have been warped by family prejudice during his developmental years. There are families that live in a state of constant depression, of martyrdom and of continuous self-punishment. A child in such a family is taught over and over again that life is really miserable and that misery is the richest experience of living. By adolescence, the child in this family will be chronically depressed—and depressing.

There are many reasons why a family neurosis starts, but this way of life continues because it has become protective and rewarding for the family. In the neurotic family, the members maintain and perpetuate the neurosis. It is impossible for a child to grow up in a neurotic family without himself becoming neurotic in some way because to be nonneurotic in this kind of family would make the other family members anxious, angry and rejecting.

Edward sought psychiatric consultation when he was was 19 years old because he was "always unhappy." He said that he "did not fit in anywhere."

Edward is the eldest son of Lithuanian Jewish parents who survived years of Nazi persecution in Europe before they emigrated to the United States. The family comes from a small, strongly orthodox Jewish sect. Since coming to the United States, the parents have had to work very hard in menial, poorly paying jobs in order to scrape out a marginal, meager existence. With good reason they have felt that the world has been against them. They have been persecuted viciously. They have always been part of a small social minority group, subject to constant attack and ridicule. They have raised their son in the belief that he must never trust other people—never.

Now Edward has started in college. As he moves out into the big world outside his family, he senses that he has never been able to trust anyone. He has no friends —not even his parents. He does not know how things happen in this world—this world outside his very small inwardly directed family circle. Over the years he has been taught never to trust and therefore, even though he would like to trust, he does not know exactly what trust is. He wants help in some way, but he has learned through his childhood that everyone who helps ends up hurting—this his parents have told him again and again. He wants to be understood, but his mother and his father have taught him that he must always keep distant from "them," from those people who could understand. It would be easier for Edward now to withdraw into his own private, suspicious world, but he wants to grow emotionally and intellectually. He would like to share in the world that he sees around him. He realizes that something is wrong. He comes for help.

These teenage patients often come for evaluation or treatment when the neurotic patterns of behavior that they have learned in the neurotic family cause stress and conflict with the nonneurotic people they meet in their day-to-day activities.

Jim was the only child of two professional parents. He was 17 years old. His only sister had died when he was 3 months old. When he was 5 years of age he had a near-fatal throat infection. During his school years he has been plagued with recurrent asthmatic attacks.

Both parents have been very careful about their son's health. Jim's father made sure that his son took all the cold medications. His mother knitted a neck protector to wear when he had a cold. Jim was teased unmercifully in school because of this protector. During Jim's childhood his parents taught him not to go out into the cold, not to take part in rough games, not to get his feet wet. Like his parents he has taken laxatives routinely for his bowels, antacids for his stomach, aspirin for headaches and, of course, his daily asthma medication just to make certain that he did not have an asthmatic attack.

When Jim was in his senior high-school year, he began to be increasingly depressed. Eventually, two days before Christmas, he swallowed 30 of his mother's barbiturate pills and had to be hospitalized. During his hospital stay he asked to see a psychiatrist. With no prompting, Jim talked for almost 2 hours about his feelings of dissatisfaction, despair and emptiness. He felt that somehow he had been "cheated." He knew he had missed out on many things, but could not understand why this had happened to him. He sensed that something was wrong "somewhere." He felt vaguely that he should change. He wanted to work on "his problem" and he wanted guidance in doing something.

That evening, after this interview, Jim's mother and father descended on him. They brought him a thick sweater because he "must be cold" in that hospital room. His mother had cooked some special delicacies for him because she "knew" the hospital food "must upset his stomach." Both parents reassured him that everything would be all right at school because his father had talked to the school principal. By next morning, Jim no longer wanted to work on his "problem." He sat listlessly in the chair by his bed and said vaguely, hopelessly, "What's the use?" He had no will to talk about anything now. "It's just the way things are, I guess." And Jim went home to be part of his family.

In a family where the family way of life is psychotic, the children are almost obliged to grow up psychotic. These families live in their own private world, reacting to each other and to the world around in their own idiosyncratic fashion. By adolescence, a child in this family will have made the family psychosis his way of life and he too will be firmly psychotic. During his developmental years his psychotic way of adaptation will have been constantly reinforced. To be nonpsychotic in the psychotic family the youngster would have to be "sick." If he has any ability to relate meaningfully, he will have learned in his relationship with his parents to be like they are. If the family members are psychotically aggressive, paranoidal, suicidal, or delusional, the child in such a family will grow up with these behavior patterns.

Many ethnic and cultural groups will tend to perpetuate certain neurotic or psychotic family traits. If a family is part of a persecuted minority group, they and the other members of their community will naturally be uncertain and suspicious. Even when the social reasons for this suspiciousness are reduced or removed, the cultural attitudes will long continue. If a community is raised in the strong belief in hellfire, damnation, and a righteous, vengeful God, a family pattern of depression, self-punishment and rigid conformity will be accentuated and maintained by the social customs. If the child comes from an ethnic group in which violence is an acceptable way of living, he will tend to be violent even when he goes out into a nonviolent society. In evaluating the disturbed teenager, members of the professional team must measure whether he can give up his neurosis or his psychosis; they must know whether he can change or whether any change means that he will have to give up his family, his culture and his community.

Often the neurotic or psychotic behavior of the adolescent is supported by what he sees and hears in the general world around him, in that world that is supposed to be healthy. Why should he control his murderous aggressive impulses that some people are calling sick when he can see men, women and children butchered everyday on television on the newscasts or during the evening entertainment? Why should he change his suspicious attitude when speaker after speaker on the television screen rants about being victimized? Why should be trust anyone when he is told constantly by leaders of his community that "they" are not worthy of trust? Why should he control his impulses to enjoy himself now when billboards, magazines, and television all urge him to have his pleasure now and pay later? He can watch and he can listen to angry, bitter and aggressive men and women flaunt their lack of self-control and judgment for a tolerant, almost encouraging national audience. In the newspapers he can read how the good, the kind and the hopeful are cut down, ravaged and destroyed—with impunity and sometimes with social approval. So very often in his everyday living the teenager—healthy, neurotic or psychotic—is taught new forms of sick behavior by a society that is supposed to be healthy. The sickness of society, the sickness of the family and the sickness of the adolescent may all complement and perpetuate each other.

When the neurosis or the psychosis of the teenager is part of his family neurosis or psychosis, usually he is brought for evaluation or for treatment only when his behavior has been disturbing to people outside his family or when the adolescent himself has been disturbed by the contrasts and conflicts he now faces. As the adolescent moves away from his family, he may find to his dismay that the family way of life he considered so good and productive is unacceptable to the wider community outside his family. He may be sent for evaluation by this community because the behavior he learned from his family is intolerable in general society. In evaluating any adolescent, his way of life must be evaluated against the usual patterns of his family and his culture. It may be unreasonable to ask him to change a life style. If he became "healthy" in the ways of "normal" society, he might make this change only at the price of becoming intolerable to his own family or to his own community. By adolescence the personality patterns are relatively established for most people. These behavior patterns can still be modified but they cannot usually be totally removed. The disturbed adolescent from the disturbed family may be helped to change his way of life so that he produces less anger and less anxiety around him in the supposedly nonpsychotic, nonneurotic world, but it may be unreasonable and indeed impossible to expect him to change his basic personality structure.

THE DEVIANT CHILD GROWN UP

There are some adolescents who have grown up "different" or deviant from other members of their family and their community. Some of these children are different because constitutionally they were born with different sensitivities and capabilities. Some children are different because they meet with different responses from the people who care for them. Most deviant children develop their different patterns of growth because constitutional predisposing factors and environmental forces interact and lead to different ways of adaptation.

Warm, emotionally normal families may have children who are born with little interest or ability to relate to people; constitutionally these children are predisposed to be autistic and they never do emerge from their own private emotional world. Other children are born with a normal ability to relate but, because of constitutional hypersensitivity or unusual sensitivities or because of pervasive environmental rejection or confusion, never do develop their innate ability to relate meaningfully. Such children grow up increasingly idiosyncratic and autistic. Children who are autistic, whatever the cause, may be socially and mentally retarded by adolescence or may present a wide range of psychotic and neurotic symptoms.

Autism in adolescence most commonly arises from other causes that are frequently missed. Children who have a normal emotional capacity to relate to other people, but who must grow up in a world that is different because of a perceptual handicap, may come for treatment or evaluation because of behavior that appears to be neurotic or psychotic. These children perceive their world differently because their way of perception is different—

they are the blind, the deaf, the retarded. As they have developed, they could only respond to the world around them on the basis of their own perceptions, but these perceptions have been different from the commonly accepted ones. Their different way of perceiving forces them to develop different patterns of thinking and reacting. If their perceptive ability has been very different from the usual ways of perceiving, the world they see and the world they react to will be markedly different from what is normally experienced. Even though these children may have been born with a normal ability to relate and to feel emotionally, they will have no option but to grow up in their own private world. In adolescence they will present a picture of symptomatic autism, with many neurotic and psychotic-like symptoms.

The child who is born deaf or severely hard of hearing does not learn to use sound to communicate or to form his thinking. His thought patterns are based more on smell, feel and sight. He reacts to people according to the vibrations he senses from them. He responds to the emotions he sees in their eyes. His behavior may appear unusual, neurotic or psychotic, to "normal" people. The blind child lives in a world without color or visual form. He has to learn appearance of people around him by their sounds, by the softness of their face and by their smell. Black power. Black sin. Black of night. What can "black" mean to a blind child? The blind adolescent perceives differently and has to work out his way of living according to his perceptions. To a blind teenager, an egg may be like molasses because it is sticky when it is uncooked, or like rubber when it is cooked—because that blind adolescent may know an egg by the touch and the feel. The retarded child grows up seeing people doing and saying things that he does not completely understand in their terms and so he has to explain these things to himself by his measures. He may tell time by the expression on his teacher's face—she always is tired by 2:00—or by the emptiness of his stomach, while "normal" children tell time by the clock.

In adolescence, these children may be brought for evaluation because they are different and their different attitudes and behavior may bother people. The health professional must make the diagnosis in these adolescents very carefully to learn whether there are constitutional or environmental factors that have forced them to grow up perceiving the world differently and made them react to this world on the basis of their own different perceptions.

DRUG-INDUCED NEUROSES AND PSYCHOSES

In recent years an increasing number of adolescents have been brought for evaluation and for treatment because they have been taking drugs. The problems of these adolescents must be considered very carefully because not only has drug abuse become an increasing problem but also it is now the acceptable social reason for obtaining treatment for a disturbed adolescent. It is easier for the adolescent and his family to seek help because of "drug abuse" rather than to ask assistance for emotional difficulties. With many adolescents and their families, drug abuse is only a small part of a much deeper, more pervasive psychologic disturbance.

TREATMENT

If it is decided that the disturbed adolescent requires treatment, the evaluation process has really only begun. At all stages of a therapeutic program, the treatment procedures must be planned to meet the needs of the teenager at a specific time. The adolescent has an ability to grow and to change very rapidly. In the treatment alliance with the adolescent, treating personnel must be constantly evaluating the youngster so that they can give him the help and the support he wants and can use at a specific moment. Most often treatment is disrupted because the adolescent has moved in his emotional development while the treatment personnel have retained the way of reacting that was appropriate previously.

In any treatment process, the final decision to use or not to use what is called "treatment" rests with the person who is called "the patient." If the adolescent does not wish to be treated, any attempt to force this kind of attention on him may be more destructive than it is helpful and may even perpetuate or accentuate a maladaptive behavior pattern. If the teenager does not feel emotional pain or does not wish to change, he will naturally resist any attempt to coerce him—even under the guise of treatment—and, as he resists, he may use the emotional and intellectual energy that he should be using to cope with his life stresses and to continue his emotional and intellectual growth.

At any time during the course of a treatment or evaluation process, the teenager may indicate that he has gone as far as he is willing to go or can go at that moment. If this is his definite decision, his decision must be accepted. The treating personnel really have no option but to accept the decision of the adolescent, as indeed they should accept such a decision made by any other patient. There are many factors in a teenager's life that may dictate more limited treatment goals than the treating professional team might wish. If the adolescent changes too much, he may become intolerable in his own family and he has to live in his own family until he is socially, emotionally and financially independent. He cannot live with the treatment team.

The adolescent and those professionals who are offering him help and support should all know that the teenager can come back later for further help or guidance. He can change his way of life in stages and, as the people around him adapt to his changes, he may then be able to adapt further. This process often takes time. Many adolescents are introduced to meaningful treatment during their adolescent years and then come back for more definitive psychologic help when they are more independent adults.

Too often caring-treating professionals refuse to accept the adolescent's right to be what he says he wants to be; members of the professional team work hard with the adolescent to help him make up his own mind and then, when he does make a decision, they refuse to accept what he has decided. His choice may be against their wishes and advise, but they have to accept this choice. Even if the adolescent decides to be inadequate, neurotic or psychotic, the caring professionals may have to support his decision because it may allow him to live most efficiently in the environment in which he has to continue living.

If the adolescent is never going to have real friends, it is useless for him to continue feeling the pain of loneliness, even though the treating personnel want him to face this pain; it is much more efficient emotionally for this adolescent to accept a life style of being lonely and to become a "loner," even though this goal may not be too satisfactory to his therapist. If it is apparent that, no matter how much he strives, the adolescent will never really succeed, it may be easier for him to accept the life pattern of being inadequate because by doing so he will then feel much less pain about his inadequacies. He may continue throughout life dependent, unambitious and unimaginative but he will have accepted himself and thus the misery will be less. Inadequacy may be the most efficient way of life for such an adolescent. If a teenager has tried to be accepted and has never met with acceptance, it may be more tolerable for him to believe that "they are against me" because then he will not feel the agony of rejection; he will not have to keep on trying again and again without success. If he believes that "they" are against him, he can stop trying, he can settle, he can relax. He will have peace. Even though his paranoid attitude might be considered sick, this sick behavior may be the most efficient way he has of coping.

While the task of the treatment team is to help the adolescent become most efficient in the environment in which he will have to live, sometimes the treating personnel may be able to change the teenager's environment. By working with the teenager's family, with his schoolteachers or with his employer, they may be able to reduce the stresses placed on the adolescent and to insure that his world is more predictable and reasonable. Sedatives and tranquilizers are often very useful in lowering the teenager's inner anxiety to the point where he can again manage. Drug treatment is especially useful when the adolescent's difficulties arise from constitutional hypersensitivities or are due to the upsurge of adolescent drives. In this era when drug use is widely abused, caring personnel must know the psychologic significance of any medication given to the adolescent. The medical benefit of any drug might be more than counteracted by the antisocial or delinquent meaning of such a drug to the teenager.

In dealing with any adolescent, even the profoundly neurotic or the psychotic adolescent, treatment must always be planned to strengthen the strengths that he has, to reduce the stresses that he faces to a bearable level and to offer him acceptable ways of intellectual and emotional growth. At all times in the treatment alliance, the adolescent and the caring professionals must be adapting the treatment approach to meet the youth's requirements. With the high energy level of adolescence and the strong natural drive towards independence and self-sufficiency, the adolescent can grow and change very rapidly. The task of the professional is to move with the adolescent and to provide him with the understanding, the support and the direction which he needs and can use.

REFERNCES

Beckett, P. G. S. (1965): *Adolescents Out of Step*. Wayne State University Press. Detroit.

Easson, W. M. (1969): *The Severely Disturbed Adolescent*. International Universities Press New York.

Kanner, L. (1963): Autistic disturbances of affective contact. Nerv. Child, 2:217–250.

Weiner, I. B. (1970): *Psychological Disturbance in Adolescence*. John Wiley & Sons, New York.

Chapter 7

BEHAVIOR PROBLEMS IN YOUTH

S. Jalal Shamsie

Once psychosis, severe neurosis, organic conditions and mental retardation are ruled out, most conditions in adolescence fall under the broad and ill-defined rubric of behavior problems. This heading includes all types of behavior of which society disapproves and to which parents object, and forms by far the most common cause for referral in this age group.

CLASSIFICATION OF BEHAVIOR DISORDERS

Attempts to differentiate between behavior disorders in children and adolescents lead us to varying opinions. There are those who suggest that dividing behavior problems into different types is a fruitless exercise since the period of adolescence is fluid and constantly changing. Labeling one type of behavior only interferes with our understanding of the total picture and may restrict us in our attempts to help. Others stress the need for identifying the different types of behavior problems because the treatment approach in each type is unique.

Based on data collected over a number of years, Jenkins and Cole (1964) suggest three categories: overinhibited, unsocialized aggressive, and socialized delinquent. For each category they describe a behavior pattern, a family background and a preferred treatment approach. Fish and Shapiro (1964) have another typology and in the Group for Advancement of Psychiatry (GAP) (1966) proposed classification there is no separate classification for behavior disorders, but these would probably be included in the section on Reactive Disorders and Personality Disorders.

From reviewing different classifications, and drawing upon personal clinical experience, only two divisions of behavior disorders seem justifiable. These are, first, problems of recent origin, which are reactive to severe environmental stress, and, second, problems of long duration, where there are fixed pathologic trends which have become ingrained in the personality structure. These trends are not seen by the adolescent as a source of intrapsychic distress or anxiety and may be termed ego-syntonic. Such a division seems justifiable since the prognosis and treatment plans for the two conditions are different. Reactive disorders usually respond well to family and individual psychotherapy. If the therapist succeeds in altering the environment even to a small degree the results are very gratifying.

In personality disorders, there is a long history of antisocial or asocial behavior. There may be evidence that, as early as age 6, the youth was stealing from the corner drug store. There may be a history of lying and truancy from school, and perhaps a trusting relationship between adolescent and parents was never established. Meaningful communication may never have been adequate and whatever communication existed may have completely broken down with the advent of puberty. One seldom finds serious behavior disorders in the adolescent who has free and easy communication with his parents.

In the treatment of young people with long histories of difficult behavior, once or twice weekly individual or family therapy may not be sufficient. In such cases, it may be necessary to place the adolescent in a residential setting where his behavior is under observation on a 24-hour basis since he may require milieu therapy in addition to individual and family therapy for an extended period.

A great deal of difficulty could be avoided if the adolescent is a party to the discussion and decision leading to his placement, and usually it is advisable to postpone his admission to an institution if he is unwilling. A short waiting period is a better solution to the problem of unwillingness than to deal with a hostile and negative attitude after he is admitted. A visit by the adolescent to the center where he is to be placed, and meeting the staff and other adolescents, could be very reassuring to him. Some adolescents may agree to go to such a center without argument as they also desire a change from the constant fighting at home. Others may see such a suggestion as further evidence of collusion between parents and therapist.

Every effort must be made to resist pressure from the parents who may be anxious to get the adolescent placed in a center. As far as possible all discussion regarding the need for placement should be carried out in the presence of the adolescent. The therapist should express his views openly and freely, even if it means upsetting the parents or causing temper outbursts from the teenager. If the therapist is in favor of placing the adolescent in a center he should make it clear that, although he is in favor of hospitalization for the stated reasons, he would not be a party to the youngster's being admitted against his will. This may not please the parents who feel some urgency for getting their son hospitalized. However, the adolescents who require urgent admission are few. In most instances the emergency is not real. It is more a symptom of the panic of the parents. These parents have to be told that the short-term benefit of getting the adolescent placed in a center against his will and thus providing some relief to the parents has to be weighed against losing the adolescent's trust. Therapist and parents both must recognize that, in the long run, they cannot protect the adolescent against himself, rather they are able only to help him take care of himself.

ADOLESCENT AND FAMILY

Most behavior problems in adolescents are manifestations of an on-going conflict between adolescent and family. The adolescent is caught in his struggle for identity, his conflict between his desire for autonomy and his needs of dependency. This has been identified by Erikson (1968), but what needs to be emphasized is that the search for identity by an adolescent causes a great deal of stress on parents. The constant questioning and testing, which is part of the process in which an adolescent finds out for himself what is good and what is right, become an endurance test for parents. To be constantly challenged and criticized is not easy to endure. To be continually told by someone who is completely dependent upon you for his basic needs that your marriage is a failure, your love for your wife is a deception, your success is based on fraud and that you really are not fit to live in the present world is enough to drive a parent to distraction. This holds true even for someone who is understanding and aware of the problems of adolescence.

The problem is further complicated by the constant testing of limits by the adolescent. It does not seem to matter that the limits are set after consultation with the adolescent. He wants to find out what would actually happen if he came home at one in the morning instead of midnight as agreed. This again can be an exasperating experience as one finds it hard to accept the fact that the same person who seems to have an answer to all problems on earth, and would be prepared to reorganize your entire life if given the slightest chance, is unable to accept the minimum of responsibility without argument and fuss. Most parents find this constant testing out and "so what" attitude hard to take.

The problems of being a parent of an adolescent are onerous even if one is aware of and sympathetic to his problems, but they can lead to an open conflict if one gets caught in the adolescent's struggle and starts reacting to his each move as if it is reasonable. The parent should not lose sight of the transient nature of the adolescent's feelings even though they are intense when experienced and expressed. I remember a father who broke down in tears when he described how hurt he felt when his teenage daughter told him that she hated him. His reaction oscillated between intense anger and intense guilt, "I could have clobbered her—what did I do wrong?" He was able to understand better when he was reminded that 2 weeks back she used the same expression to describe her feelings towards a girl who is now her best friend. Very often adults forget that part of being young is to experience every emotion intensely. When young, if one is sad, life is not worth living; if one is happy, then there is no problem which cannot be overcome. Someone without whom life cannot be imagined can almost be forgotten in a short while. Most feelings are experienced intensely but are transient in nature.

The problems reach a dangerous proportion when the parents are not only unable to empathize with the problems which are experienced by the teenager, but also start reacting and misinterpreting each move. This usually occurs in those parents who have never really solved their own conflicts related to independence and dependency.

When their son decides to act on his own, they see this as a challenge to their authority rather than a step towards his adulthood. They are afraid of losing all control of their child. In fact they not only foresee losing control but losing their child. They recognize, although at a subconscious level, that every move of their teenager towards autonomy and adulthood brings them closer to losing their "child." So starts the classic battle between an adolescent, seeking his identity and adulthood, and the parents, who do not wish to lose their child.

In most cases the problems start with the advent of puberty. "Mommy's little boy" and "Daddy's little girl" suddenly change from a sweet adorable child into a nightmare. The parents are suddenly told that they are not so great; in fact there is hardly anything they can do right. Their daughter is out late at night and they are worried to death. When she returns they are told that they were stupid to "wait up" for her. If they question further, then there is screaming and crying and each such outburst leads to further alienation between the adolescent and the parent. The parents feel the loss when there is no one who gives them a hug and a kiss at bedtime. Suddenly they find themselves short-changed. There are no returns. Parents are asked for more money or for the use of their car, but it is seldom that their son or daughter has any time to talk to them. They resent it and refuse to give money or car or whatever. This refusal increases the distance and further limits communication. Soon the relationship begins to deteriorate and mistrust replaces trust. Communication in any meaningful way stops. There are arguments and shouting, but neither side is listening any more. The same old phrases are repeated; attitudes become stereotyped. Father knows what his son is going to say even before he opens his mouh and the son knows that there is no point in listening to his father.

In most cases, this breakdown of communication can

be seen as the forerunner of troubles which finally bring the family to the office of a psychiatrist or to a Judge's Chamber in Juvenile Court. It is at this stage that the problem is most often brought to the attention of a mental health worker. It is important to remember that one is entering an on-going social crisis in a family. There is usually an undeclared war in progress between the teenager and his parents. As usual in such conflicts there is neither trust nor meaningful communication between the two sides. The therapist has to be extremely careful to make sure that he is entering this conflict as a mediator and a facilitator and is not seen as a reinforcement for one side. This is not always as easy to do as it appears. As in any war, each side has its weapons. The parents can cut off the allowances, stop all the privileges, and call the police, the court and the psychiatrist. The adolescent can run away, or do things which he knows will really hurt his parents. In the latter he has a large choice, and, knowing his parents, he can achieve his objective by letting his hair grow long, by smoking marijuana, by stealing, by doing poorly in school, or by being promiscuous. A girl may get pregnant to attain her objective.

It is remarkable that, in most of these cases, one discovers that the adolescent has not only committed the forbidden act, but also has made sure that his parents know it. Smiling, the teenage girl explained to her parents that she had forgotten the contraceptive pills in the bathroom, but refused to tell where she got them and for how long she has been taking them. The parents looked enraged and helpless, and the teenager sat there looking pleased. A hit had been scored. A battle had been won. Another teenager accused her mother of spying when the mother read her diary left in the living room. The diary contained a detailed account of the daughter's first experience of sexual inter-course and that part of the diary was in capital letters and underlined. The parents, coming from a very religious background, found this most revolting and used one of their own weapons by stopping her from going out in the evenings, although they knew that sexual intercourse took place in the afternoon, in their own home, while they were out visiting.

Anyone who has worked with this kind of problem can remember any number of similar examples all illustrating that to the young person it was not the act which was so important, but the effect it would have on their parents. They were all aware that it would result in reprisals from their parents, but then, in an on-going battle, one has to do whatever one can to hurt the enemy. They also realize that by their act they are escalating the war, but at the same time they indicate that no war can be brought to an end by one side.

ADOLESCENT AND THERAPIST

It is in this atmosphere of conflict that a therapist may be called upon to intervene. You, the therapist, may receive a phone call from the father, who states that he was given your name by his doctor who has highly recommended you. He is having troubles with his teenaged son, and he would like an appointment to come down with his wife so that both parents could give you all the facts. The implication is that after they have given you all the facts, you can see the teenager alone or with them, as then there would be no danger of distorting the truth, the truth being the events as the parents see them. If the therapist agrees to such an appointment at that time, the treatment is doomed to failure before it has started. The therapist has already sided with one of the partners in conflict. His neutrality becomes questionable and his role as a facilitator between two parties who have stopped trusting and talking to each other becomes impossible. His greatest asset in such a role is the trust of both parties. Once the therapist agrees to act for one party without the consent of the other he allows the other party to see him as a reinforcement, or as an ally to one party. From then on, anything he says or does would be viewed with suspicion by the teenager who is the person who has the real power to end the crisis. By giving the appointment to the father the therapist has not only lost his neutrality but has sided with the wrong party, the party who has no chance of winning, or even having peace without the cooperation of the other.

Once there is full awareness of the above situation, it is not difficult to see the therapist's role clearly, as that of a neutral person attempting to act in such a way as to establish a meaningful communication between two parties in conflict, hoping that it will lead to trust. The therapist's greatest asset is his neutrality and creditability. It is then easy to see that a request for help from one of the parties cannot be accepted. The answer to such a request would be that the teenager has to be a party to any agreement. The therapist is willing to intervene if both parties desire such intervention and both parties agree on the choice of facilitator. He will not participate unless the teenager has been informed and is willing to see the therapist, with the family. There should be no separate sessions for the parents unless approval is given by the teenager who may also wish such treatment. With these ground rules laid down, therapy can start. With treatment thus begun, progress can be rapid as the early distrust of the adolescent can be readily overcome in one or two visits, instead of the traditional ten to twenty visits.

The mistake of accepting an adolescent for treatment at the request of the parents occurs most often because psychiatrists tend to adhere to the medical model. They have an image of themselves as a doctor who cures and heals. They see the acting-out adolescent as someone who is sick, and they see no need to take the above-described precautions. The habit of diagnosing also helps to justify the intervention without the consent of the teenager. The teenager is sick with such and such disease and requires treatment, which the doctor will give. This medical model, when applied to a family crisis, leads to very poor results. To call a teenager, who runs away from home, sick, when he is trying to get away from an unbearable family situation, is to extend the medical model to its extreme. To imagine that one can cure running away by treating it as a sickness is to imagine the impossible. The situation has to be viewed as a social crisis in a family between teenager and parents. The therapist must also accept a more humble role than that of the agent who cures or treats, neither of which is possible in this situation. He must act as facilitator to encourage meaningful dialogue between the teenager and the parents.

PITFALLS IN TREATMENT

The pitfalls do not end with the onset of the treatment process. The two parties do not give up their hostile attitudes or distrust and, although the therapist may have established his neutrality, the two sides do not refrain from trying to win him over to their respective camps. The therapist has to be on his guard and remain ever-watchful. Danger lurks on both sides. The parents see the therapist as an adult whom they expect would naturally empathize with them. They feel that therapist as an adult has gone through life and has gained the same experience and wisdom as they themselves have gained, and therefore would certainly understand and appreciate their point of view. All this is never put into words, but is very much present in the interview situation if the therapist is sensitive to it. When the adolescent makes an emotional statement which contains some obvious exaggeration or distortion, the father looks at the therapist with a helpless gesture indicating "see what I have to put up with." Very often the father expects a nonverbal response, and the therapist has to watch that no nonverbal communication indicating a special relationship or understanding develops between him and the parents. There are other verbal traps set by the parents for the therapist. The parent makes a provocative statement and ends with a phrase like "you understand doctor, don't you." Here a nod from the therapist can cause an outburst from the adolescent who sees the foul play.

Another implicit component of the special relationship demanded by the parents is the unsaid message "remember, I pay your bills." This is used in many subtle ways. There is the phone call in which apology is extended for the delay in paying the bill, assurance is given that the check will be on its way, and then the casual introduction of the subject of the next family therapy appointment, indicating very gently that some help in supporting a certain attitude would be appreciated. This requires firm handling by the therapist as the payment of his bills could be used to seduce him away from his neutrality. The parents, having learned that they can to a degree control their son's behavior by controlling the financial rewards, do not mind trying it on the therapist. There has to be a clear understanding regarding the payment of bills at the start, and the teenager should be aware of all the facts. If any attempt is made to deviate from the early agreement, then this should be made known to both the parties.

There is the other situation, which arises after a number of visits in family therapy, in which the father suddenly states that he cannot afford to pay for any more visits although there has been no change in his financial situation. This usually occurs at a time when father's behavior and attitudes are under scrutiny, and very often when the adolescent's behavior is on the mend. This is father's way of expressing his anger towards the therapist for lack of support, and also, more important, an expression of the father's frustration in his inability to bring about necessary changes in his behavior, while at the same time watching his son change his behavior with relative ease. It is not surprising that one notices changes in behavior earlier in the adolescent than in the parents. Most adolescents do not expect a real change in their parents' behavior. They can accept their parent's limitations and can be generous about it. Very often an admission from the parents that their behavior and attitudes also require changes is satisfaction enough for the adolescent.

Examples illustrating how parents may attempt to win the therapist over to their side have been given in the foregoing paragraphs. On the side of the adolescent the danger lies not so much in the adolescent's success in seducing the therapist to his side, but in the therapist's identification with the adolescent. Most adolescents have an anti-establishment, and an anti-authority attitude. Most of them are critical of the status quo and support radical change. Very often the youngster decries the financial success of his parents, and denounces their materialistic and success-oriented attitude toward life. The danger lies in the fact that the therapist may find that he is in agreement with most views expressed by the adolescent. He may discover that many statements made by the adolescent are the echo of his own thoughts which he has never put into words and that his own social and political views are in harmony with the views of the adolescent. Although the therapist may not have as simplistic a view of the problems of life as the adolescent, who has a need to see things as good or bad to prevent confusion, the therapist may still be in agreement with the spirit of the statements. However, sharing the values of the adolescent and having similar sociopolitical views should not interfere with the therapist's role as facilitator between the two parties in social conflict. Neutrality is not always easy, especially if the parents tend to have sociopolitical views which are at the opposite end of the continuum from the therapist's. The therapist has to remind himself constantly that even if he agrees with the adolescent's views on the Vietnam War, this is irrelevant to his "there and then" role. That the parents do not share his sociopolitical views bears no significance to his role as facilitator. It is more than likely that both parties in the course of time will discover where the therapist's sympathies lie; however, it is important that both parties know that sharing certain views expressed by either party will not interfere with the therapist's objectivity and neutrality in his role as a facilitator.

From the time of referral to the conclusion of the treatment, the way is full of pitfalls for the professional who is trying to help a young person. In a social conflict which has gone on for some time, the therapist has to win the confidence of both parties. He has to show that he understands the problems facing the parents and at the same time point out where they may be unwittingly blocking the growth process of the adolescent. He has also to convince the youngster that although the therapist may belong to the same generation as his parents, that does not mean that he inevitably supports their views. It has to be pointed out to the adolescent that his demands for more autonomy are not justifiable when his behavior shows an inability to accept responsibility. Most adolescents accept controls when they feel that their needs are understood. They also accept responsibility when they feel that they have been consulted. This desire to be a person, rather than "Daddy's little boy," makes it necessary that they be presented with the problem, and included in the search for a solution.

REFERENCES

Erikson, E. H. (1968): *Identity: Youth and Crisis*. W. W. Norton Co., New York.

Fish, B., and Shapiro, T. (1964): A descriptive typology of children's psychiatric disorders: II: A behavioural classification. In: *Child Psychiatry, Psychiatric Research Report # 18*, October. R. L. Jenkins and J. O. Cole, Eds. American Psychiatric Association.

Group for Advancement of Psychiatry (1966): *Psychopathological Disorders in Childhood: Theoretical Considerations and a Proposed Classification.* Vol. VI, Report No. 62, June.

Jenkins, R. L., and Cole, J. O., Eds. (1964): *Child Psychiatry, Psychiatric Research Report # 18,* October. American Psychiatric Association.

Chapter 8

OUT-PATIENT THERAPY WITH YOUTH

Donald J. Holmes

Traditional psychiatric thinking about various mental and emotional disorders has been dominated for the past century or so by what has recently become popularized as the "medical model of mental illness." Our colleagues in clinical psychology and psychiatric social work seem particularly eager to remind us of the inapplicability of certain classical medical approaches (to patently physical disease) when they are brought to bear upon a host of psychologic disturbances having no demonstrable cause-and-effect relationship with genetic, neurophysiologic, metabolic or other clearly defined disorder of bodily functioning.

Instead of taking up the cudgel for Mother Medicine, however tempting that may be, it should prove more fruitful simply to acknowledge that in certain important respects the objection to this so-called medical model of mental illness seems indisputably valid. This viewpoint spuriously implies that in mental illness, as in physical illness, there is a discrete and tangible etiologic agent which produces a disease syndrome—a complex of more or less uniform manifestations known as "signs and symptoms." Also implied by it is the promise of a specific therapeutic remedy for the malady, some pharmaceutical or other precise medical technique which heals by eradicating or neutralizing the causal agent.

This is actually how it works in the kinds of mental illness (febrile delirium, for example) which are secondary to some patently physical cause, such as an acute bacterial septicemia, in which appropriate antibiotic therapy overwhelms the offending agent and thereby relieves the mental manifestations of the illness.

This arrangement, however, accounts for only a small percentage of the total mental and emotional symptoms that psychologic clinicians of whatever persuasion are called upon to deal with. In the bulk of them the causal "agent" is plural rather than singular, and these, as a rule, are also less palpable and thus less amenable to physical demonstration and manipulation.

Even so, the official psychiatric nomenclature for such disorders, by means of the terms and phrasing used, strongly suggests that the impact of disequilibrating life stresses typically produces a uniform, pathologic strain response which can be relieved at once by such "specific therapy" as tranquilizing medication or insight-producing psychotherapy. By the subtle conversion of simile to metaphor the latter appear to become scientific medical fact and are thus the more conveniently retained within the medical dominion.

CHANGING CONCEPTS OF PSYCHOPATHOLOGY

Whether it is intended or not, terms such as "psychoneurosis," types one, two and three, tend to preserve a conception of psychologic disturbance as an endogenous, physically based disease response, the cause of which is to be located straightway within that hypothetical but quite nonexistent anatomic locus of the personality known as the "psyche." The patient is counted mentally ill not so much because of what is happening to him to make him that way, but because of what he is like to begin with— a "neurotically predisposed" or "latently psychotic" individual whose intrinsic "disease" is merely released, or precipitated, by some passing external stress to which the rest of us are by nature immune.

Granting that there are certain inherent and early acquired differences between people in their ability to withstand one kind of circumstantial stress or another, it nevertheless remains that the vast majority of psychiatric patients who come to us for service are suffering principally from the pressure of circumstances which are, in reality, extremely hostile to their total well-being. They are not so much sick in their bodies as they are troubled in their lives and they are mentally ill only in the sense that one can become profoundly depressed by the loss of a loved one, chronically furious about the beatings he regularly receives from a brutal father, or sickened to the point of frozen immobility under the influence of a mother who secures her hold on a growing child by fostering in him a welter of undeserved guilt feelings.

It may also be granted that a fair measure of temporary, symptomatic relief can be accorded the person who is suffering this kind of pain by offering him certain easily administered palliatives, and to be sure there are many times when this is the best therapy available. Even then, however, it is hard to escape the feeling that we are only giving opium to a man who is being torn on the rack, when we would much prefer to strike his chains that he might walk away from his bed of torture a free man.

Of the many alleged mental disease entities that we have been schooled to recognize, the most damning of all is that known as "schizophrenia," or the "schizophrenias." In its time the concept did yeoman service in helping to rescue the deeply troubled and disenfranchised from the totally condemning implications of its diagnostic predecessor, "dementia praecox," which in its own time and turn had served well by saving these individuals from the floggings, flames and shackles of the demonologists (Zilboorg, 1941). But now having done its duty it is hopefully going the way of its obsolete, nosologic antecedents, as it has long since become a clinically futile, even destructive, substitute for understanding. It is a vast wastebasket of a "diagnosis" which now functions chiefly as an easy expedient for the clinician who is either too busy, too disinterested or too ill-informed to set about learning more about what forces are actually bringing his patient to grief.

Here it is not opportune to submit a detailed case against the existing system of psychiatric nomenclature (Holmes, 1972). For now it is enough to note that its principal victims have been those of "low caste" who for one reason or another have also been declared mentally ill: racial, national and other ethnic minorities, the poor and the young. These account for all but a small percentage of our "schizophrenics," as we who do the diagnosing are much inclined to reserve the nicer appelations (adjustment reaction of adult life, acute depressive reaction, etc.) for ourselves and for our more prosperous and politically advantaged cohorts of like station (Hollingshead and Redlich, 1958).

Similar objections must be leveled against the class of disturbances presently known as "personality disorder," in which a person's behavior, rather than painful psychologic symptoms, provides the criteria by which the alleged mental illness is identified and specified. In making such a pronouncement, more often than not the culturally cloistered diagnostician is simply expressing his personal disapproval of some other person's way of life—of his way of making a living, of dealing with a heavy-handed authority that has singled him out for the scapegoat's role, of his preference for some statistical variant in sexual gratification, or of his electing to exercise his natural right to choose his own poison.

These are extremely treacherous standards upon which to construct a judgment that the person who has come to you (or been referred to you) for help is, in fact, mentally ill. Perhaps the clinician's surest safeguard against the damage that always lies potential in this brand of judgmentalism is a principle of ethical practice that is at least as old as medicine itself, which is the primacy of patient service. We are available but we do not intrude— we do not seek to sell our services lest our motives be suspect.

Most of the people we see may in some sense and to some extent be "in trouble with themselves," but when their living circumstances are carefully examined and well understood it will be found in most cases that the lion's share of their distress arises from the people and the conditions they are trying to live with. The clinician's central task, then, is not to brand his employer with a nasty name of his own devising, but rather to take whatever reasonable measures he can to assist his client to serve himself better amidst "the slings and arrows of outraged fortune" that plague and beset him.

Where adolescents and youth are concerned, especially during the past 10 years, it has grown more and more difficult to decide where the greater fault lies when the young person and his society run afoul of each other. The well-publicized nuclear threat and ecologic crisis, the dismayingly dogged persistence of racial discrimination, the ever-widening economic gap between the Haves and the Have-nots, and, perhaps most discouraging of all, the steady growth of strong government and publicly sanctioned, gestapo-like law enforcement—all are present in profusion for the young to deal with.

If the young are not always philosophically temperate in the face of these crushing concerns, if at times they lash out in crude and technically illegal ways, and if there are intervals when they find the pain too great to endure without the restorative consolation that drugs can sometimes offer, then perhaps we cannot only understand them, but even admit that they may not be, by virtue of age and innocence alone, entirely wrong. Our commitment is to help them as *they* would be helped and not as we believe they should be helped.

THE TREATMENT AGREEMENT

This primary allegiance to one's client is easily enough honored when the client is an economically independent, self-contained and socially conforming adult who pays his own fee, breaks no laws and does not contest the professional authority of his therapist too hotly. It is apt to be quite otherwise, however, when the client in question is a suspicious, querulous adolescent who comes for his "therapy" as if he were visiting a probation officer and very often at the behest of parents or parent-like agencies (school, juvenile court, or the like) who have made it painfully clear that they consider him sick in the head and in the most urgent need of a heroic personality revision at the hands of of the awesome "headshrinker."

This negative set is generally complicated by the fact that the fee for service is being paid by the referring complainant, who cannot help but hope that the "revisions" to be made will accord with his own expectations and not with those of the identified "patient." A good therapist will, of course, attempt to serve both masters as well as possible (or give the devil his due?), but when a conflict of interests develops, as it usually does, then he must almost always resolve it *in favor of the person he has been retained to serve*. This is not really so much because it is the medically ethical thing to do, but because it is the only way that works.

The question most often heard in this connection: "Yes, but what if the therapist knows that his adolescent patient is going to harm himself? Doesn't he owe it to all concerned to inform the parents so that they can take steps to protect him?" The answer to this is a resounding "No," and for two rather obvious reasons. To do so would violate the client's right to confidentiality, a right which must be strictly respected if a trusting relationship is to develop. Second, the presumption that the parents or surrogates would be able to supply protection against the self-injuring behavior is usually unfounded.

A third pitfall in the argument that such violation of privilege is sometimes justified resides in the capriciousness of such expressions as "the patient will harm himself" or that he is practicing "self-destructive behavior." This can be a most difficult determination to make. As a rule it is just a harried adult's way of saying that his adolescent daughter may have become sexually active or is "taking dope." These behaviors may obviously be injurious but are not inevitably so, as when the girl is adequately protected against unwanted pregnancy, or is smoking several marijuana cigarettes a week instead of swilling cheap wine and driving her car at high speeds while under its influence.

Ideally, the young patient will come to regard his therapist as an interested and companionable ally in virtually all things, though also a ready and able disputant on any point at issue between them. If the boy is stealing or "doing drugs," our first concern is that he not be caught, leaving the stealing and drug use to be reckoned with in due time. If the girl is sexually active we would first help her to avoid pregnancy, and if she should contract syphilis we arrange for appropriate treatment without betraying her to anyone who would use this information against her. At times we even frankly conspire with the boy to protect him from the consequences of his own inclinations to inordinate honesty, especially when he is dealing with a law that has grown too muscular, too intrusive, too controlling and constrictive.

> Sixteen-year-old Hank was hauled into juvenile court on a charge of possessing and vending marijuana, having been entrapped into the supposed offense by an overzealous police officer who accomplished his mission by masquerading as a "hip" adult in dire need of a joint. Partly because Hank was white, and also because his father was a person of some stature in the community, the juvenile court judge considered settling the charges informally after having a long, heart-to-heart talk with the boy in the privacy of his chambers.
>
> On the day before this judicial therapy was to take place, Hank came to my office to confer about what dangers he might anticipate in the encounter. The most likely of these was that the judge might decide to forgive and forget (exact no additional penalties) *if* Hank would confess the error of his ways and promise never to do it again. He was extremely anxious about the temptation to deliver the expected lie in order to keep himself out of reform school, but had almost resolved to take the risk. I was successful in dissuading him from this course, however, by reminding him of Machiavelli's sage counsel—to the effect that promises made under duress need not be honored—and by citing his Constitutional right to refrain from giving any injurious testimony against himself.

When the young patient is dealt with in this spirit there is rarely any serious problem about his keeping his out-patient appointments and profiting from them. Having good reason to regard his therapist as a good and reliable "Vergilian friend" (Masserman, 1969) he comes to talk with him not because he has to but because he wants to—

although he will seldom acknowledge this in so many words.

SOME COMMON PSYCHIATRIC SYNDROMES OF OUR TIME AND PLACE

A mentally ill person, by one definition (LaBarre, 1954), is anyone who falls conspicuously out of step with the other people around him. Should he somehow manage to convert his idiosyncrasy into profit or prestige he becomes known as gifted, talented, or an "exceptional" person, but otherwise the odds favor his being considered mentally ill by his community and probably by himself as well.

That which we call "mental illness" is necessarily and inevitably culture-bound. Many of the formulations constructed during the past half century or so to explain various psychoneurotic and psychotic reactions, in psychologic terms, have depended for their authenticity on a prevalence of certain communal attitudes that have generally denied the individual an opportunity to express openly a variety of largely inherent drive propensities not of his own choosing. The chronic frustration resulting from the prohibition, according to these now classical formulations, mobilizes one or several *mental mechanisms of defense* which subserve the general purpose of warding off a fully conscious awareness that such drives are even present (Freud, 1946). These mechanisms, though they mask the drives from consciousness, do not eliminate them, and a variety of possible psychologic symptoms (anxiety, depression, irrational guilt feeling, obsessional rumination, etc.) are the consequences of this defensive inefficiency.

In actual practice we have been much inclined to behave and speak as though we believe that the defensive operations should be strengthened and the drives they defend against diminished or eliminated. How pleasant and uncomplicated it would be if only we could dismiss such an unphysiologic proposition as nonsensical and unnecessary, but this, unfortunately, is no more justified today than it has ever been. Instead we find that we are simply continuing to move in the direction of a compromise that allows for greater freedom of tender, loving and non-injurious sexual expression ("make love") while imposing even more stringent taboos against those behaviors classed as aggressive, hostile, alienating ("not war").

This is perhaps the most useful generalization to be drawn from the enormous body of psychologic theory that we are accustomed to dealing with, particularly when we are bent on establishing fresher and more meaningful indices of "psychopathology" in a dynamically changing culture. The "classical Freudian neuroses" still exist, of course, but as mass norms of thinking and behavior change in the direction of freer personal expression, those symptom reactions stemming from severe social proscriptions of the sexual, for example, will steadily diminish. More and more of our adolescents and youth are little if at all troubled by the frankly conscious deliberation and "acting out" of drives that, a generation ago, would have been the seed for a shattering panic attack or a florid paranoid psychosis. Many of these young people converse casually about their masturbation, isosexuality or ambisexuality, voyeurism and exhibitionism, transvestism, sexual relationships with parents and siblings and group sexual encounters as if they were reflecting aloud on a weekend of skiing or about how many servings they had at last evening's ice cream social. These subjects are usually introduced not as complaints in themselves, but only as incidental to some other presenting complaint—usually having to do with an immediate and current, emotionally critical transaction with some other person or persons.

Thus, rather than trying to *name* specific pathologic states, as if they were indeed eternal and immutable psychologic diseases, it should be much more worthwhile simply to describe several of the commoner syndromes of our time—but only after acknowledging that these too will change as the social influences necessary to their development wax, wane and vary in quality.

Culture Shock Phenomena

This very state of accelerated social flux increases both the quantity and quality of stress to which a person may find himself subjected as he moves from one community, with its own characteristic and usually well-entrenched standards and superstitions, into another and substantially different one.

Susan, 18 years of age, was referred with the diagnosis of "acute schizophrenic reaction, catatonic type" by her college counselor and with a recommendation for hospital admission and protracted, inpatient treatment.

At the time of my first meeting with Susan she was virtually immobilized by anxiety, guilt and self-condemnatory feelings. Her conversation was limited almost entirely to brief and all but identical sentence fragments having to with her worthlessness and the futility of her situation.

Her story was commonplace. She had been born and reared in a small midwestern town. In this setting, instantaneous obedience to parents was automatic, twice a week church attendance compulsory, strict curbs against peer socialization were in force and she had little reason to challenge the assumption of her parents and neighbors that she would "finish school, settle down, get married, have children" and live out her remaining 50 odd years of life in foreordained domestic bliss.

Throughout childhood and most of her adolescence she had been a model child and had accepted the community's version of her destiny as good, proper and unalterable. But she was intelligent, observant, thoughtful, and was not only exposed to television but, had friends who had traveled farther abroad than she had from the old home town. She had already concluded that her parents and all of the older neighbors who had gone the route prescribed for her seemed to have had all the experiences ordained for her except the bliss. She completed high school with honors, but it was at about this time that she began to realize, however dimly at first, that she wanted something better than the midwestern small-town life for herself.

Her symptomatic response began within several weeks after she entered the small, Protestant college that her parents had selected for her. Although she felt that the courses presented no serious challenge to her abilities, she soon found that she was unable to study, attend classes, go to meals or converse with her classmates. She spent almost all of her waking hours sitting in a chair in her room, staring at a wall. Her thinking rapidly tightened down to the one or two sparse themes she was able to confide during her first visit with me.

It would not be feasible here to detail the events that led to her gradual but steady improvement over the next two years. However, through psychotherapy, she was carefully and tactfully exposed to what can only be called religious reeducation. In this, her mind was largely disabused of the punishing, peeping Tom "god-in-the-sky" imagery that had loomed threateningly above her since earliest childhood and of the terrifying conviction that she would quite literally burn in hell in retribution for the anger and resentment that she felt toward her parents and for the compelling stirrings that she was only then beginning to sense within herself.

Over a matter of months, through talks with me and with the help of some suggested reading, she learned painfully but eagerly about her own body, and she learned also to experience, name, and come to agreeable terms with the drives that dwelt within her. With some encouragement she got a job as a waitress (having dropped out of school prior to her first visit with me) and made a deliberate effort to expand her social life. Within six months she was feeling well enough to return to school, but this time to a college of her own choosing, a more open-minded and easy-going one than the first. After a successful year there, and encouragement from me, she transferred to a large and quite liberal state university.

In this instance it would seem reasonable to propose that Susan became ill because she unconsciously sensed that her living circumstances were intolerable to her and that she would remain ill until she found her way into conditions that would make it possible for her to return to life. My task, in essence, was to identify this need, help her to clarify it in some detail in her own mind and to reinforce her efforts to make the therapeutic transition.

Susan's experience might also serve well to illustrate another common syndrome of our time and place.

Identity Crisis

Thanks to public-school education and the mass media, Erik Erikson's thinking about "identity" and "role diffusion" has taken a firm hold on the popular mind (Erikson, 1950). So much so at the college level, in fact, that the very terms have come to serve as an oft-heard complaint.

Indecision about future plans, whether about one's love life or choice of tasks, is a notorious mischief maker and it is terribly important that the person who is temporarily caught in the throes of this kind of life crisis not be misidentified as "mentally ill." At times it is only through the natural desire to "beef up" our own professional role and to enhance our personal self-esteem that we inadvertently make theoretical mountains out of ordinary molehills, then proceed to worsen our client's condition by seducing him into elaborate, elegant-sounding and nigh interminable "therapeutic programs" that often turn out to have quite the opposite effect from that intended.

Authority Conflict

The issue of widespread youthful rebellion has long since become one of popular interest and concern. As implied earlier, when due allowance is made for the social context in which certain types of "antisocial behavior" occur it is no longer reasonable for the psychotherapist to dismiss his rebellious young patient, out of hand, as a "personality disorder" or "delinquent character neurotic."

In human history, youthful revolt and revolting youth (and it must be confessed that they are not always altogether lovable) have always performed a vital service in the civilizing process, first by identifying and publicizing crying social deficiencies and then by relentlessly badgering their elder power incumbents into instituting the necessary remedies. Their steadfast position against racial and religious discrimination, despotism in the courts, munitions research and military training in the universities, compulsory military service in a war that is not of their own choosing, the martial abuse of small, weak nations by large and powerful ones and glaring economic inequities both domestic and international—these can hardly be discounted as the psychotic ideation of an epidemic paranoia.

The familiar arguments against youths' occasional readiness to take recourse to violence are firmly based on an amazingly lopsided definition, or conception, of the term "violence." When a local sheriff completely shaves the hair from the heads of peacefully protesting students his action is said to be nonviolent, but when the students try to resist a police assault against them their self-defense is called violent. When a full-grown man of sound mind and vigorous opinions is sentenced to 10 years in the penitentiary (without chance of parole or appeal) nominally for the possession of two marijuana cigarettes, but actually because he is a long-haired political dissident, then his imprisonment is called nonviolent. When high-school honor students are denied the right to attend school because someone has decided that their hair is too long or skirts too short, this, too, is called nonviolent. When a handful of priests and nuns, true to their calling, arrange to put a crimp in the operating capacities of the most powerful military organization the world has ever known by blowing up—not its people but a few of its heating ducts—this is also called violent. But when flaming napalm is sprayed across helpless women and children in Southeast Asia, the action is justified as a tactical prophylaxis against an even worse counter-violence. When black men are denied opportunity and held in contempt by their white neighbors and they object to this and urge their colleagues to fight back, they are called militantly violent. But when they are shot to death in their own beds, this is called law enforcement.

Not long ago I received an urgent phone call from the mother of a 15-year-old boy whom I'd seen as an out-patient on several occasions, this time with the complaint that "he's in his room sobbing and smashing his fist into the wall, and threatening to take his .22 rifle and shoot the first pig (police officer) he finds."

Joe had first been referred to me by his parents because of irregular school attendance, poor grades, and because he was associating with the "street people and radical student faction" on a nearby campus. During our several conversations it was immediately evident that he was a very intelligent, dynamic youngster whose school difficulties were due ostensibly to the now familiar complaints against our public education system: "a treadmill for sheep," "irrelevant," "a laundromat for establishment brainwashing," and so on. He fell in with the older, radical students because he was in deep sympathy with their views, and he articulated his defense of these views far more logically than the average "rebellious youth" of his age would be able to do.

The emergency call from his mother had been prompted by an incident of that same morning. Joe had been talking with his best friend, a student activist in his early twenties and a regular contributor to one of the local underground newspapers, when a group of policemen entered the friend's room, without a warrant, assaulted him physically and carried him off to jail without informing him of the charges against him (theft of several hundred dollars worth of small arms from a federal depot) or advising him of his right to counsel.

When Joe arrived home, furious and in tears, his mother urged him to call me for an appointment to come in and "talk it over." Although he liked and respected me, he declined the advice on this occasion because a psychiatric consultation under these conditions would be tantamount to an admission that his emotional reaction was irrational, immature—neurotically determined. I concurred with his decision and suggested to his mother that she try to convey to him a two-part message from me. First, that there are better and worse police officers and that a random shooting might mean the death not only of a good man but of a potential friend and ally as well. (When I later discussed this with a politically involved young attorney friend he smiled brightly and volunteered: "I could give him a list!" But his offer was not accepted.) Second, that such an action might bring him the dubious satisfaction of vengeance fulfilled and ephemeral martyrdom via the press, but that if he really wanted to help the cause he would be far better off to stay his anger, sharpen his thinking and writing skills and find that ultimately the pen is indeed mightier than the sword at accomplishing desperately needed social change.

The next day his mother called to say that Joe had accepted this advice. A calculated risk was clearly taken in this management, but even now it seems a vastly superior alternative to the solution which might come first to mind— involuntary hospitalization by court order on the grounds that the boy was "mentally ill" and potentially dangerous to others.

In psychiatric circles a favored dynamic formulation concerning the origins of adolescent rebelliousness is that the rebelliousness represents nothing more than the neurotic, transference-like displacement—to society at large—of angry and retaliatory feelings engendered in the adolescent's relationship with his parents and therefore irrational, unrealistic and "sick." What this formulation neglects is that the parents may in fact be exemplary representatives of an increasingly oppressive and authoritarian society and that the youth's revolt against his parents is as reasonable as it is against society.

Whatever one's political orientation, the surest guideline in matters like this is more medical than political. Physicians, or any other clinicians in the helping professions, are not the hirelings of some great, faceless and monolithic society, but the responsible agents of individuals who come to them for help. And the person who argues that a physician must also be a good citizen may be reminded that he can best do that by being, first and foremost, as good a physician as possible.

Drug Use

This is another headline topic of our time and place, but it is also most germane to any clinician's workaday practice with youths.

Ideally, no human being would ever need to take a drug for mood improvement, "mind expansion," or for any other reason. But as in most things concerned with human beings, the actual falls considerably short of the ideal. Man has always needed and used his various soporifics and stimulants and will undoubtedly go on doing so into the unforseeable future. Thus, the question is not whether drugs will be used, but about who shall decide which persons of what age and under what conditions shall use what drugs. Expressed personally, the question would be posed this way: "Whom will I accept to decide for me what drugs I may or may not take?" In quality it is about that same issue as that involved in the censorship of ideas: "Whom will I accept to decide what books I shall read and which movies I shall be permitted to see?" The answer, of course, is: "No one! These matters I would much prefer to decide for myself—that I shall insist on deciding for myself."

There are hopefully not too many people who would contest this position seriously—when it is taken by a solid, upright citizen who is a thoroughly solidified pillar of the community. But what about the young people—the ignorant and the inexperienced—must they not be protected from the potentially catastrophic consequences of their own poor judgment? About some things, of course, but about a great many others most emphatically "no." The most obstinately abiding attitude of elders toward the learning capacities and adaptive resiliency of their young is one of incredible, almost killing condescension.

> During a brief vacation a few months ago I sat with a friend on the veranda of his cottage, chatting, admiring the beauty of the lake, and thoroughly enjoying a before dinner drink. As our respective adolescent children were also present the conversation turned quite naturally to the subject of drugs. My friend was uncompromising in his vehemently voiced conviction that "drug abuse" was a certain sign of "weakness, moral decay and deterioration of character in the youth of our day."
>
> After hearing him out I smiled generously, touched my glass full of bourbon to his glass full of bourbon and replied: "I'll drink to that."
>
> He nodded blankly and resumed his diatribe against the youth "drug culture" with full force, when his adolescent

son suddenly interrupted with a plea to me: "Wait a minute! Do that again, please. He didn't even get the point!"

He didn't, and he wouldn't—perhaps he couldn't.

All of us, it seems, are constantly surrounded by people who are not only passionately willing to make decisions for us, but who will imperiously insist on the right to do so. There have been and still are many places where the existing order of things has given the people the power to enforce this perverse wish, but those who make and enforce laws in the face of today's generational schism are gradually learning that even though they are still able to inflict immense suffering on those who would choose for themselves, they do not, in fact, have enough power to fully impose their will upon others.

> Not long ago, at the suggestion of a mutual friend, I met with a candidate for high public office to discuss the "youth problem," with particular reference to psychotropic drug usage. In order to lend some reality to the encounter I arranged to have two university students, one 19 and the other 20 years old, present for the discussion.
>
> At one point in the course of a lively conversation my esteemed guest remarked: "We don't want to make drugs like this available to them because we're afraid it will interfere with their productivity."
>
> In response to this one of the students leaned forward, quite incredulous: "But Mr. (candidate) if you will give either of us the money, we can be back here in half an hour with almost any amount of any kind of drug you can think of and at a reasonable price."
>
> "Well," he answered after a moment of reflection, "at least it's not being offered for sale in the stores."
>
> To this I replied: "No, not in our stores, but it is all in abundant supply in *their* stores."

Although the multimillion-dollar, underground drug industry is controlled at the top by experienced and well-established old Crime Syndicates, most of the lower echelon distribution and retail merchandising is in the hands of adolescents and youths who are practicing free commercial enterprise with wondrous abandon. The main governmental thrust to curtail this traffic is directed at the small retailer and the consumer, as they are easy to detect, prosecute and persecute. Failure to legalize this commerce deprives us of an opportunity to: (1) reap an enormous revenue from taxation and (2) set and enforce high standards of quality control for direly needed consumer protection.

A certain small percentage of young drug users are suffering from authentic, highly personal forms of mental illness, as is also true for some of us who are veteran members of the booze, tranquilizer and pep-pill generation. But neurosis does not explain most of the extremely extensive use of marijuana and other nonaddictive, euphorogenic or mildly hallucinogenic drugs by millions of young people who are clearly destined to become tomorrow's establishment.

For an explanation of this phenomenon we must look to a social rather than an individual "neurosis." The most conspicuous offender in this regard—a sharply intensifying atmosphere of authoritarian oppressiveness at every level of our society from federal government to family—has already been referred to. Thus, to impose additional strictures upon young people who are mostly seeking to alleviate the symptoms of social and political suffocation is very much like administering an oral arsenic preparation to a patient who is already suffering from chronic arsenic intoxication. The harder we fight it, or the more vigorously we "treat" it, the worse it gets.

Looking at the problem in this light, the clinician may better understand that there is no justification whatever for taking a critical, forbidding, or condemnatory attitude toward the young client who is using drugs. As a rule, I simply listen to the youth's experiences with as much interest as I can muster, while attempting to draw him out as much as possible on the other, more positive and creative aspects of his life. I do not hesitate to let him know when he is boring me to tears with his endless recitations of his various highs, lows, "bummers," and of his petty and usually unprofitable drug transactions. Nor am I loath to scoff a little at his readiness to accept pharmacologic dosages in terms of "hits" and "caps," or to shake my head sadly when he uses cute little popsicle names to describe potions that may—as far as he knows—contain anything from starch to strychnine.

Education, gentle persuasion and an occasional touch of good-natured cajolery have long been the most effective agents for helping the clinician to treat his clients, and this is as true now as ever. It is heartwarming, it should be added, to see how well most youths respond to this receptive, even appreciative attitude toward their struggling efforts to come to some workable terms with their very difficult and complicated lives.

Sexual Relationship Disturbances

Once again, our conceptions about the normal and the abnormal sexuality in human relationships must undergo a certain recalibration as we take note of the striking changes that have taken place in the climate of custom over the past decade or two. The customary categories of psychologic disturbance most affected by these changes are, in broad terms, those concerned with the contractual details in the relationships between men and women (or boys and girls), and more specifically with those behaviors that have heretofore been designated without question as pathologic "sexual perversions." The import of these palpable changes to the youth culture must be painstakingly appreciated if the younger members of our clientele are to be received sensibly and helpfully.

Perhaps most of us, during our own "formative years," were warned repeatedly by our elders against marrying someone only because he was charming, handsome, a "peachy" dancer and a good "makeout artist." The members of the generation following us are extending the principle one step farther: don't marry someone just because he's a "good lay." In their attempt to go about the spouse-choosing business with greater care they are waiting longer before choosing, in order to test out in advance the finer character attributes of a prospective mate by associating with him longer and more intimately and by associating with more prospects before making any choice at all. They seem to be realizing that almost everyone in the world is a "good lay," that sexual attraction in itself is a notoriously fickle and unstable basis for an enduring and satisfying, long-term relationship ("marriage"), and that people must have many more lines of camaraderie and communication than sex if they are to have much chance of success in this historically tangled and troubled liaison.

During the past 50 years or so, psychiatry has devoted much effort toward inducing people to discriminate more carefully between their erotic and aggressive strivings, and to favor the former over the latter in their actual behaviors. The next 50 years may well find us encouraging a similar, more exacting distinction between our erotic and affectional (agape) strivings. In the rising generations there is already a discernible trend in this direction. The male and the female, the black and the white, the Jew and the Christian perceive each other more sensitively and treat each other more considerately than was true in the days of our youth. Many of them no longer speak of mistresses, lovers and affairs, because the kinds of misogynistic relationships thus designated are falling out of existence in their community. Steadily replacing them is the *sexual friendship,* in which it is pretty much taken for granted that if two (or even more) people meet, like and respect each other and can reach a reasonable prior agreement about the terms of their relationship, that they will naturally and by mutual consent proceed to enjoy each other to the fullest. The advent of effective, easily available contraception has not seriously affected the "morals" of the young, but it has drastically altered our communal judgment about precisely which behaviors are now to be considered more or less moral.

Hence, our conventional deliberations about "promiscuity," "perversion" and "adultery" are giving way to a more timely understanding of this aspect of moral, or "healthy," human behavior. The dictionary reminds us that "promiscuous" refers to that which is haphazard, random, ill-considered and pointless. There is a substantial difference, in other words, between being promiscuous and having many friends. Nor does it make much sense to apply these older standards to the young couple who have formalized their intention to live in a long-term, binary relationship chiefly for mutual aid and companionship, with some understanding beforehand (though usually not enough, it must be admitted) that their agreement does not preclude the possibility of some future, mutually enjoyable and life-enriching relationships separately, with others.

With all of this there has been a wholesome downgrading of the importance of sexuality in interpersonal relationships generally, and thereby much less need for the enormously magnified, obsessional, frustrating and time-consuming ruminations about it which have been such a familiar and rather terrible part of our own experience. Accompanying this is an equally healthy degradation of the infamous double standard of sexual morality, a vigorous surge in the age-old movement toward social and economic equality for women, and a striking increase in socially sanctioned bisexuality. Any busy and experienced psychiatric clinician today has surely learned by now that extremely few of the bisexual, isophilic or other "para-philia prone" persons passing within his professional purview are suffering from mental illness in any clinically significant sense of that phrase.

But rapid social metamorphosis of this sort is never without some disturbing reverberations emanating from the grinding fault between the old and the new. Two major and frequently encountered problems of transition here are: (1) premature, self-imposed typecasting by young people who—because the power of the old taboos has not been entirely dissipated—are all too ready to declare themselves consummately "homosexual" at the first tick-ling of an isophilic urge, and then to dedicate themselves to fulfilling every detail of this arbitrary social role as they have been reared to understand it, and usually without giving themselves half a chance to branch out toward a broader and perhaps more rewarding variety of experience: (2) a growing fear of heterosexual inadequacy in young men who have some reason to question their ability to measure up to the expectations of their womanly counterparts, who are no longer as willing as they have been to conceal the reach of their desire or to forego a more fulfilling male response to it. It seems beyond question that the women's liberation movement, the spirit of which is far more inclusive than the several action groups officially espous-ing it, is taking a certain toll from the masculine sexual potential. Anatomically and physiologically, woman is immeasurably more potent than man, and when the latter is no longer able to preserve the ancient illusion that he is an all-knowing and all-powerful superstud in relation to her—that he is really no match for the drive and endurance of a healthy woman—then it is hardly surprising that what little he has becomes even less.

As this awareness grows, women will obviously have some serious choosing to do. More of them will probably turn to a fuller and somewhat different kind of sexual satisfaction with other women, which indeed a great many seem to be doing already. Those who still want men may be willing to continue with some of the old affectations of ignorance, innocence, and politely feigned admiration for her partner's peerlessly priapistic penile prowess, in order not to frighten him with too challenging a display of her sexual superiority.

An individual's right to make this kind of choice is the helping clinician's prime consideration. In my own practice I have found the problems presented by two women who are "married" to each other, or by two men who are similarly related, to be virtually identical to those complained of by the conventionally married heterosexual couple. For the most part, these problems are best dealt with by the same quality of acceptance, interest, and pragmatic problem-solving approach that would usually be exercised in more run-of-the-mill marital counseling.

Any thorough discussion of more exact clinical approaches to such specific disturbances as frank impotence, genuine "frigidity" (actually a rare condition, as most of that which is so called is really secondary to masculine incompetence, ignorance or indifference), voyeurism, exhibitionism and other "paraphilia" could easily fill a volume or more. Most to be emphasized here is one point of ethics and one of technique.

1. There are few things more futile than undertaking to *treat medically* a condition that is *not a disease,* but a way of life. If one man finds his pleasure in strolling the boulevard with lace panties and brassiere beneath his gray flannel suit and does not complain of it, then it is not ours to thrust upon him a gratuitous and denigrating judgment disguised as a medical diagnosis, nor to offer uninvited "treatment."

2. Traditional psychotherapy, for the person who earnestly wishes to enlarge his sexual horizons, has enjoyed an extensive field trial over the past several

decades and been found seriously wanting. More recent approaches to behavior therapy which rely upon the alternate administration of viands of volts, depending upon whether the "patient" arouses and responds with the right stimulus or the wrong one, seem little more promising. However, a carefully controlled, planful involvement with a considerate, well-informed, sensitively communicating and otherwise well-qualified clinical assistant (C.R.T., for comprehensive relationship therapist in prefence to "sex therapist") is giving some cause for at least tentative optimism. Along with a few other clinicians in the field of human relationships, I have cautiously undertaken a sort of modified "tea and empathy" approach to some of the problems under consideration—but only for those who sincerely desire and actively request such changes for themselves and who have given free consent after having been thoroughly informed about the attached conditions. A detailed discussion of this subject is not in order here, and for that the interested reader is referred elsewhere (Holmes, 1972).

PSYCHOTHERAPY

Even though the earlier section titles of this chapter have referred to changing concepts of psychopathology, common syndromes of our time, and so on, the dominant theme of these discussions has been psychotherapy throughout. There is surely little to be gained by concluding with a warmed-over dissertation on the customary measures and influences of therapy which are already well known to anyone trained in psychiatry, clinical psychology, psychiatric social work, the ministry, or other branches of the helping professions. More to the point for present purposes will be a concise, selective critique of certain of the livelier issues in the field of youth therapy today.

Drug Adjuncts

Except for convulsive disorders, certain other organic brain syndromes and severe psychotic states, drug therapy has limited value as an adjunctive treatment for adolescents and youth (if only because they are already doing a bit too much of it on their own, as mentioned earlier). The short-term use of mild sedation is justified during times of acute emotional turmoil, but more than this is seldom indicated. More and more psychiatrists are beginning to share the not altogether unfounded youthful suspicion that drugs are too often used for the purpose of quelling rebelliousness, or to alter thinking in some covertly prescribed direction—a sort of hypnotic with a purpose that would not necessarily be to the recipient's liking.

Format and Setting of Therapy

Therapy is no longer to be conceived of as a strictly formal process which takes place in a fancy office, with "patient" on a couch or bolt upright in a chair, free associating endlessly (if indeed it is possible to find one who will even agree to try this) while oracular therapist sits, stone faced and immobile, behind a massive desk doing his majestic headshrinker thing.

Probably the commonest and most damaging misconception abroad in contemporary youth therapy has resulted from the epaminondic misapplication of the psychoanalytic model of therapy to the modern setting and clientele, which require far more activity than passivity. There are still many occasions that call for quiet listening, but even this should be done actively and accompanied by active thinking that points toward an eventual response. There is also still an occasional need for catharsis and abreaction (to talk it out, get if off one's chest, or work it through), and for the clarification and interpretation of internal experience and overt behavior, but the younger the other person the greater will be his need for thoughtful feedback about himself. Perhaps what he needs most of all is a chance to structure his sometimes rather amorphous and turbulent experience into articulate thought, that he may better perceive its form and rely upon it with greater assurance for future direction.

The Treatment Relationship

In the course of developing what is usually spoken of as a therapeutic relationship, shared feelings of fondness and closeness commonly develop quite apart from any prior intention or design on the part of either participant (or group member) and something should be said about both the role and the threat of this quality of intimacy in the treatment relationship. This is undoubtedly the most delicate matter of the many we must routinely deal with, but because it is there in reality it must be dealt with, and to this it should be quickly added that deliberation does not necessarily constitute advocacy. The fact remains, even so, that old taboos against emotional closeness, against touching ("physical contact") and against even fuller relatedness are falling away in actual practice. For now it might be enough to say that when a therapist stiffens and retreats from a young girl's spontaneous expression of affection or appreciation, his shrinking response—by betraying his own fear of his deepest feelings toward her— might well frighten her far more than would a relaxed and casual acceptance of her heartfelt gesture. This is not a therapeutic "technique" that can be measured out and dispensed in divided doses, and it is obviously not without some considerable risk of dreadfully antitherapeutic complications.

However defined, therapy consists far more of attitudes than of technical operations, of real, immediate and personal interaction than of any bag of tricky techniques or self-conscious, quasi-scientific procedures. The relationship that develops in the course of it is far more real than "neurotically transferred," and much that is swept beneath the rug of transference serves chiefly the therapist's need to protect himself from recognizing this.

> A 20-year-old student was referred by her gynecologist because of a relatively minor complaint which he felt was beyond his competence: "I can't seem to find a boy I like well enough, and respect enough, to enjoy a complete relationship with . . . you know . . . including sex. Here I am practically a grown woman and still a virgin—I guess that's pretty abnormal these days."
> I assured her that in my opinion, at least, it was not at all abnormal. As we talked more about it, it came out unmistakably that her own explanation of her disinclination to "go the whole route" was essentially sufficient in itself. She was a very intelligent and attractive young woman who valued herself highly and she was simply not willing to settle for any fast, easy bargains in her relationships with others.
> On her fourth visit she began to express some positive feelings for me, and in such candid and literal terms that I wondered if she might not be falling into the role of "patient in therapy must fall in love with doctor if neurosis is to be resolved." I asked her if she had come across the concept of "transference" during any of her undergraduate work. Se replied that she had heard the term but was uncertain about its meaning. I briefly explained it to her and after a moment of thoughtful reflection she answered:
> "I see how that could be, but it's certainly not the only possible explanation. After all, you're a man and I'm a woman, so it's in us and in the situation. Feelings like that don't *have* to be transferred from anywhere. I could have those kinds of feelings toward you if I'd never had a father or a brother—or if I'd never even met a man before."

The preferred language of psychotherapy is nontechnical, the language of the shops, streets and campuses. No words, no ideas are forbidden in this realm. In today's youth community such ancient shockers as "fuck," "shit," "tits" and the like are used quite conversationally by our finest young people, not so much to shock as to undo the superstitious sanctification of language that has permeated past custom. Among adolescents and youth the language fads change so rapidly that the "in" argot of yesterday will be quite passé today and herein lies a trap for the over-straining therapist who would effect total peership with his young clients. They enjoy their own play with words and phrases, but they are also deeply respectful of the "king's English," as long as it transmits clear, straight thinking about things that really matter to them.

Certain golden rules of child-rearing may also be applied with good effect in the therapeutic relationship. If the therapist is not in some good measure enjoying what his young clients are doing and saying, then the odds are very great that it is he, not they, who is suffering from some distortion of viewpoint. And on the perenially difficult question of how to foster a good relationship, it would be difficult to improve on the attitude of the wise parent who understands that the harder you hold on to them the farther they move away and the more you let them go the closer they stay.

The much vaunted aggressiveness and seductiveness of the young patient is probably much exaggerated in our usual discussions about them and more often than not our complaints on this score are chiefly our own projections. The young person who is treated honestly, fairly and amiably rarely if ever becomes either verbally or physically abusive. The "seductive" girl can scarcely be this way all by herself—there must be a "seducee" to name her as "seductress," and we must wonder why he would make such an issue of so declaring her. Shortly before his death several years ago the wonderful Dr. Henricus Rumke, while serving as discussant at a conference on "The Seductive

Patient," surged forward to the podium, waving his arms and laughing: "What is so wrong about being seductive? Please, try to seduce me—it would be a very nice compliment. I like it!"

Other Aims and Services in Therapy

That which we call psychotherapy is as often as not a sort of intensive, nonauthoritarian tutorial activity, in which the therapist functions variously as catalyst, counselor, confidant, source of information, and part-time defense attorney. With patients (clients, students, or whatever they choose to be called) the last-named function is by no means the least. A youth therapist is frequently called upon to represent his young employer's interest in the most anguished disputes with parents, school, law-enforcement agencies, the military and others. Strangely and rather sadly, there is little if anything in our various psychologic schools of thought to guide us in any practical way in our efforts to arbitrate and adjudicate these contests, some of which seem quite petty and others great.

Over the years, while groping about for some reliable standard of reference to direct me in mediating these motley antagonisms, I have found myself turning time and again, almost automatically, to a most curious but extremely helpful code of reference. The common parental complaint that "he's a pathologic liar," when carefully researched, usually turns out to mean that the youngster has lied to survive while being unduly pressured to give self-incriminating testimony. At other times we learn that he is being found guilty without having an opportunity to face his accusers ("Never mind who told me—I know what you've been doing!").

"He's been reading filthy, obscene books and magazines" is another garden-variety complaint, but when the prosecuting parent is asked how he came by the evidence, we find that the harassed defendant has been the victim of unwarranted search and seizure. "I forbid him to associate with that gang of hippies" is a denial of the right to lawful assembly and the outraged demand that long locks be shorn and all drugs eschewed is in violation of the guarantee of "Life, Liberty and the Pursuit of Happiness."

However odd it may sound at first, the legal principles explicit in the American Constitution, and particularly in the Bill of Rights, provide more practical and applicable pointers for child-rearing and for the conduct of therapy, than do all of our technical treatises put together. The accused is innocent until clear proof of his guilt is in evidence. He is entitled to an impartial hearing in an adversary setting ("Don't you talk back to me!"). There shall be no cruel and unusual punishments ("You're an hour late—you're grounded for a month!"). The accused may not be required to testify against himself ("Stop that lying and be honest with me—you've been doing it, haven't you!?").

Today, hundreds of thousands of adolescents and youths have seceded from hearth and home and are on the road, too early and with too little to support them. Having been denied their heritage of liberty at home they are taking recourse to yet another and slightly older precedent: "That to secure these rights, Governments are instituted among Men, deriving their just powers from the consent of the governed. . . That whenever any Form of Government becomes destructive of these ends, it is the Right of the People to alter or abolish it, and to institute new Government." Youth are also people, and those of us who are telling them to love America or leave it never seem to specify which America we mean—Patrick Henry's or the Pentagon's.

Freedom, like fascism, begins at home and the prophets of doom who blame the ills of youth on "permissiveness" are only adding to the fires of oppression that are driving them from us. Our great freedom charters were indeed written to permit the "flowering of human eccentricity" (Douglas, 1970), and it is our repudiation of this principle, our fear-inspired denunciation of all that is in the least novel or spirited that stands as the severest mental and emotional disorder of our time.

Those of us who relate ourselves to the young in any fashion at all that is intended to be "psychotherapeutic" must understand these things, or we will be of no value to them whatever. Their argument is with the despot, not the sage. They are not antagonistic to old people, but to old thinking, congealed opinion, and to simple bigotry in everyday life. If we do not offer better than this we shall surely lose them, and they us.

REFERENCES

Douglas, W. (1970): *Points of Rebellion*, Random House, New York.
Erikson, E. H. (1950): *Childhood and Society*, W. W. Norton Co., New York.
Freud, A. (1946): *The Ego and the Mechanisms of Defense*. International Universities Press, New York.
Hollingshead, A. B., and Redlich, F. C. (1958): *Social Class and Mental Illness: A Community Study*. John Wiley & Sons, Inc., New York.
Holmes, D. J. (1972): *Man and His Mind*. Little, Brown & Co., Boston.
LaBarre, W. (1954): *The Human Animal*. The University of Chicago Press, Chicago.
Masserman, J. (1969): Personal communication.
Zilboorg, G. (1941): *A History of Medical Psychology*. W. W. Norton & Co., New York.

Chapter 9

IN-PATIENT TREATMENT: THE FIRST FIVE YEARS OF AN ADOLESCENT UNIT

S. Jalal Shamsie

In recent years an increasing number of adolescents are being referred to hospitals and clinics. This increase can be partly explained by a relative increase of young people in total population, and partly by an increasing interest of professionals in the problems of the young. It is not clear whether there has been an actual increase in the incidence of emotional problems in adolescents; however, greater efforts have been made in developing programs at both in-patient and out-patient levels to meet the rising number of referrals.

Concern has also been expressed regarding the quality of these programs and the training of the personnel involved, as evidenced by the position statement of the American Psychiatric Association (1967) and the editorial entitled *Adolescent Psychiatry* appearing in the Canadian Medical Association Journal (1967).

In the late fifties, such an increase was observed in the number of adolescents referred and admitted to Douglas

Hospital, a 1600-bed psychiatric hospital located 3 miles southwest of Montreal, serving the English population of the province of Quebec.

Serious problems involving adolescent treatment on adult psychiatric wards in the Hospital were also recognized when this increase occurred. Although adolescents admitted with psychotic illnesses presented few problems when treated with adults, most of whon were also suffering from similar breakdowns; problems especially arose when adolescents with severe behavior disorders were treated with adult patients.

These difficulties could be partly attributed to the ward program on most of the adult units at the Hospital, which was more oriented toward the management of psychotic patients. The aggressive, demanding and manipulative behavior of the adolescents with behavior problems put a great strain on the small number of staff available. This strain usually resulted in the rejection of these adolescents by the ward staff, which often led to their transfer to another ward, where a similar pattern was repeated. This movement of the adolescents from ward to ward resulted in a worsening of their behavior and, consequently, increased rejection by the staff.

In order to solve these problems of treatment of behavior-problem adolescents, as well as to deal with the increasing number of adolescent referrals, it was proposed that an adolescent unit be developed in a building especially designed for this purpose. It was hoped that by establishing such a unit (1) it would be possible to develop a program which would be suitable to the needs of adolescents, and (2) the adult wards could be freed from disturbances caused by patients in this age group.

Other considerations such as research, training of personnel and teaching, which would result from such a program on an adolescent unit, were also important; however, the primary motivations which led to the establishment of the unit were the two given above.

Some adolescent units were already in existence outside Canada at that time, and other adolescent treatment centers have also been set up since the development of the adolescent unit at the Douglas Hospital. There are, therefore, a few accounts available in literature which describe the development of an adolescent unit (Cameron, 1953; Hendrickson and Holmes, 1959; Kohlmeyer and Rafferty, 1966; Warren, 1953), but the admission policy and the experimental approach adopted at the Adolescent Unit of Douglas Hospital do seem to have been somewhat unique, so as to warrant an analysis of its first five years.

In this chapter, emphasis has been placed on describing all the approaches and techniques employed in the running of the new adolescent unit, those that were successful as well as those that were not, in the belief that the reader will benefit from such a discussion and perhaps avoid some of the pitfalls described herein.

The adolescent unit was started in 1963 in a new building located on its own grounds, as part of the Douglas Hospital. The unit, designed for adolescent treatment, had a capacity of 18 beds, 9 beds in each wing of the building with the central portion of the building housing such facilities as occupational therapy, school and dining areas.

The staff included one full-time psychiatrist, one resident psychiatrist, one social worker, one psychologist, one occupational therapist and one teacher. There were 18 psychiatric nursing assistants and one registered nurse acting as head nurse.

It was decided preferably to admit adolescents with serious behavior problems. This decision was made partly because of the problems encountered with their management on adult wards as described earlier. But other considerations were also involved and some of them were:

1. To provide an active treatment unit for these adolescents. At that time there was no facility providing active treatment for adolescents with behavior problems. The level of care in the correctional institutions where the

majority of adolescents were being treated was extremely low, with no professional staff available; these institutions were providing food and shelter, but little in terms of programming.

2. It was considered that by moving into the field of treatment of behavior-problem adolescents, which had been neglected heretofore by professionals, an interest could be created which could lead to an upgrading of existing facilities and opening of new ones.*

3. It was recognized that an 18-bed unit could not in itself fulfill the needs of the community for the treatment of adolescents with behavior problems. However, it was felt that the unit could be an essential link in a chain of facilities.

Adolescents with behavior problems included the three types described by Jenkins and Hewitt (1944) and by Jenkins (1962)—the overinhibited, the unsocialized aggressive and the socialized delinquent. The chronic psychotic, the brain-damaged and the mentally retarded adolescents were considered unsuitable for admission. It was felt that the needs of these youths would be so radically different from the needs of adolescents with behavior problems that it would be unwise to treat them in the same milieu. Youths having acute psychotic breakdown and

---

*This hope has largely been realized in the development of a clinic in 1966 as a result of the involvement and efforts of the staff at the adolescent unit at Douglas Hospital. The clinic was located in the building of the Juvenile Court to provide assessment and interim treatment to all youths referred by the court (Child and Family Clinic, 1966). The establishment of this clinic, besides reducing the waiting period for psychiatric assessment from 2 to 3 months to 1 to 2 weeks, has provided coordination between the court and receiving agencies.

Indirectly, because the staff of the court clinic visited and evaluated treatment centers, its establishment has also resulted in general improvement in the level of adolescent treatment at other centers.

These developments serve to illustrate that the decision to admit behavior-problem adolescents, besides providing direct help to those admitted, has indirectly helped the facilities in the community looking after such adolescents.

those in other emergency states were admitted on short-term basis.

The question of admitting members of both sexes was considered. Although the physical layout was such that it was possible to admit both boys and girls, it was decided to admit either girls or boys, as it was feared that there would be enough problems with 18 behavior-problem adolescents under one roof without adding the stimulation which would result from the proximity of the two sexes. The wisdom of this decision is now questioned as at present there are 9 boys and 9 girls in the same building. However, this change came only after 5 years when the unit had become stabilized and staff members had gained experience. Whether in its early stages the unit would have survived with acting-out boys next to promiscuous girls is open to question.

After it was agreed that members of one sex only would be admitted, it was decided to admit girls in the vain hope that they would be less difficult to control than boys. This expectation proved to be wrong, as our later experiences with a boys' unit showed that girls were, in fact, more difficult to manage.

For the sake of presentation, the 5-year period (1963–1968) seems to fall into four phases. In each phase the special problems confronted are described and the steps taken at that time to meet those problems are outlined. Under the heading "On Reflection," in each phase there is a discussion of how things could be done differently, as viewed by experience and hindsight.

PHASE I (6 MONTHS)
A QUESTION OF SURVIVAL

Problems

Although the number of patients cared for in the first 6 months never exceeded 10, and the staff-patient ratio during the day was one to one, the level of disturbance in the unit was very high. There were physical attacks on staff members and damage to the property.

Each patient was expected to follow the program which was drawn up for her one week in advance. This program consisted of school, occupational therapy (O.T.), sewing, cooking, and other group activities. Each patient had psychotherapy twice a week. There was also group therapy once a week. The families of all the patients were seen and whenever possible family therapy was undertaken by the therapist. In the evening, patients were encouraged to organize their own program with the help of the staff.

The patients exhibited a great deal of reluctance in attending the programs. At every step there was resistance and an attitude of "what are you going to do about it?" Any pressure from the staff resulted in a confrontation, with a great deal of open hostility.

Steps Taken

On the assumption that the hostility of the patients was related to anxiety and insecurity as well as lack of knowledge and experience on the part of the staff members, meetings were held at the end of each nursing shift. All staff members present attended these meetings. The incidents were reviewed and the cause of each and its handling were discussed. In the hope of providing support to the staff the Director was present in the unit from morning until late in the evening. He often attended the 11 P.M. meeting of the nursing staff at the end of the evening shift. He was also available by telephone on an almost 24-hour basis, and returned to the unit whenever a crisis occurred or his presence was requested.

A special teaching program was developed for the nursing staff. Each Saturday morning a meeting was held which lasted 3 hours. The program consisted of a seminar, providing theoretical considerations and a review of literature. In the second part of the program there was a discussion on the state of the unit. This program was carried out by the Director of the unit with the help of the psychologist and was continued on a weekly basis for a period of 6 months. The majority of nursing staff attended this program, including those who were off duty, without any remuneration.

On Reflection

It is felt that at the opening of an adolescent unit there should be at least one senior staff who has had the experience of working with adolescents.

Guidelines and rules regarding the behavior of the patients should be established before the unit is started. Patients should know the types of behavior which are not acceptable and would lead to loss of privileges. Since it was decided that no rules should be established unless their need has been clearly expressed and felt by the staff, these guidelines were not provided.

Some of the anxiety of the staff was related to the extremely hostile attitude of the members of the adult services staff, whose attitude was understandable since the adolescent unit appeared as a privileged and favored child. The unit was located in a new building with ample space; there was more than one-to-one staff-patient ratio in the unit—higher than that in any other part of the hospital —and some of the best staff members from other parts of the hospital had asked if they might join the unit. Also, the value of the unit was questioned by the members of adult services staff because of the type of patients who were admitted: those who appeared to behave more like spoiled kids than "sick" teenagers. Administration also expressed concern and criticism when the acting-out behavior of the patients led to destruction of the property. The staff of the unit felt caught between the hostile and critical attitude of the staff of the hospital and the verbal and physical aggression of the patients.

It is felt that some of the above-described difficulties could have been avoided if the staff of the hospital had been consulted regarding the need for establishing an adolescent unit. Because the establishment of such a unit has an impact on all related facilities, the hospital staff should be consulted and oriented toward some of the problems which could be expected to arise in the early operation of such a unit.

PHASE II (12 MONTHS) A PERIOD OF EXPERIMENTATION

Problems

In the first 6 months of this phase, on the assumption that the extreme hostility of the patients might be related in part to the staff's insistence on attending the program, and restrictions regarding leaving the unit, it was proposed and agreed upon by the staff that, for a trial period of 6 months, no pressure be put on patients regarding attending the program. Patients were also told that they could leave the unit after informing the nursing staff. These changes resulted in the following problems.

Although the level of aggression was somewhat reduced, the program was unattended. Patients spent most of their time in their bedrooms, or watching television, and hardly anyone appeared for school, O.T., or other activities.

The patients would leave the unit, and sometimes not return for a few days. When they returned they looked tired, exhausted, and slept and rested most of the time. They would seldom discuss with the staff members the experiences they had had while outside the unit. Once recovered from their fatigue they would take off again. It was recognized by the staff that the unit was being used as a hotel, with patients leaving whenever they liked and returning when they felt the need for food and shelter.

Steps Taken

It was concluded after 6 months that a liberal approach of this kind was unworkable with this group of patients. After a review and discussion with the staff it was decided to lock the doors of the unit. It was also decided that to control the aggressive behavior of the patient, drugs would comprise the main therapeutic tool. Each patient had a written p.r.n. order to be used when, in the judgment of the nurse, the patient became unmanageable.

On Reflection

The liberal approach which characterized the first 6 months of this phase appeared to have little therapeutic value for this type of patient. Most of them had a fragmented super-ego and hardly any inner controls. The permissive approach did not add to the strengthening of their inner controls. The socialized delinquents saw the situation as one where they could use the unit without the unit making any demands on them. This experience for them was hardly any different from their staying downtown with a group of "delinquent" friends. It is conceivable that the liberal approach might be useful with a group of overinhibited adolescents.

In the second half of this phase, drugs were the main therapeutic tool and the unit was closed. Although this approach made the staff feel more secure, its usefulness in modifying the behavior on a long-term basis is questionable. Drugs were seen by the patient as a hostile reaction of the staff in spite of verbal statements from the staff to the contrary. The use of drugs as a control measure led to deterioration of the relationship between staff and patients.

The pharmalogic efficacy of the drugs (phenothiazines, chlordiazepoxide and diazepam) in controlling aggressive behavior in these patients is also questionable. In most cases, large doses of drugs had to be used to control aggressive behavior effectively, but the use of this heavy dosage resulted in patients being unable to participate in the program or psychotherapy. When the dosage was reduced or use of the drug discontinued, there was no change from the original behavior. On the whole, phenothiazines were found to be more useful than other anti-anxiety drugs in controlling aggressivity.

PHASE III (18 MONTHS) A PERIOD OF STABILIZATION

During this period, from the experience of the past 18 months, certain rules and regulations were developed. The unit was once again opened, with the understanding that patients could not leave the grounds without permission. If they did leave without permission, on their return they were confined to their rooms until an understanding was gained regarding the reasons for leaving, their experiences when they were away, and their present feelings.

The program was made compulsory and if a patient did not appear for any part of the program she was expected to stay in her room for that period of time. It was decided that all aggressive behavior would lead to loss of privileges. In practice, physical aggression invariably led to loss of privilege. If hospital property was destroyed, the patients responsible contributed a sum of money from their allowances as compensation. These rules were discussed and explained to the patients before being enforced.

During this period, tension in the unit was relatively low. The number of aggressive acts was markedly reduced; in fact the unit became a fairly quiet place with most patients attending the program. Each patient continued to be seen in psychotherapy twice a week and in group therapy once a week. Patients were seen with their families in the evening.

Problem

The only outstanding problem during this relatively quiet period was occasional group acting-out, which took the form of taking drugs, indulging in homosexual behavior or scratching the wrist.

Steps Taken

The acting-out usually provoked a strong reaction from the staff. Most of its members had strong feelings regarding such group behavior. They were helped to understand that this type of action represents a mechanism calculated to arouse staff anxiety. It was suggested that the staff members should make it known, without showing undue concern or anxiety, that they do not approve of such behavior. Most of these fads disappeared when little notice was taken of them.

PHASE IV (2 YEARS) A FOLLOW-UP STUDY AND A CHANGE IN PHILOSOPHY

After the unit had been in operation for 3 years, it was decided to make a follow-up study on all patients who had left the unit, to evaluate the effectiveness of treatment. The method adopted will not be described here, but will be the subject of another publication (Shamsie, in process).

The patients who were rated as improved and who attributed their improvement to their stay in the unit were asked, "What in the unit helped you most?" Most patients assigned their improvement to the help received from the nursing staff. Others mentioned other patients in the unit as the source of help. Psychiatrist, social workers and psychologists who were conducting formal individual psychotherapy were seldom mentioned.

The results of this follow-up study were discussed by the staff.

There was general acceptance that the patients spent most of their time either with other patients or with the nursing staff, and that there was a great deal of therapeutic potential in these two groups. Individual psychotherapy for 2 hours a week was considered insufficient. It was recognized that it was not possible to provide more time than this for individual psychotherapy with the staff available. There was also the question as to whether individual psychotherapy was the ideal treatment approach for adolescents with such long-standing personality disorders. It was decided to use the therapeutic community approach as outlined by Maxwell Jones (1968) with some modifications. It was hoped that this would make it possible to use the therapeutic potential of the nursing staff and patient population on a formal basis.

In introducing this approach it was decided to discontinue individual psychotherapy. Patients were divided into three groups, with a therapist assigned to each group. Two therapists were psychiatrists and one was a social worker. The groups met for an hour, 4 days a week. Members of the nursing staff were similarly divided into three groups, each group being directly responsible for a patient group. The nursing staff of the relevant group attended the group therapy meetings.

The highlight in this approach was the daily morning meeting which was held at 9 A.M. and lasted for an hour. The meeting was attended by all staff members and patients. For the first 6 months it was chaired by a staff member, later by an elected patient representative. At the meetings the incidents that had taken place in the preceding 24 hours were discussed and decisions were made regarding the steps needed to be taken in view of the developments. At times the staff members disagreed among themselves in discussing a problem. However, it was felt that disagreement among them, in a meeting with patients, had therapeutic value. The patients had a great deal of difficulty in dealing with disagreements either among themselves or with authority figures. They would often resort to swearing, leaving the room, banging the door and actually hitting the person who disagreed with them. An honest disagreement among the staff, which could lead either to one person seeing the other's point of view, finding a compromise, or even agreeing to disagree, would be a live demonstration of how staff deals with disagreements. To avoid disagreement in a meeting with patients would amount to pretending that the staff do not disagree.

Problems

There was resistance from the staff in accepting the breakdown of hierarchy, and allowing the patients to participate fully in the decision-making process. Although the approach was explained and fully accepted by the staff there was resistance from different groups when the mechanics of it affected them. For example, although the nursing staff accepted the approach they were reluctant to discuss the nursing report in the morning meeting. Similarly, although the psychiatrists were keen to adopt this approach they were resistant to the idea that the group in the morning meeting might decide on all requests from patients, such as whether or not the patient should go downtown.

The staff had great difficulty in fully participating in the morning meeting. There was always the tendency to discuss the problem with a patient or a staff member on an individual basis.

Steps Taken

This approach was introduced after discussion with staff and patients at all levels extending over a period of 5 months.

On Reflection

On looking back over the 5-year period, it appears that the therapeutic community approach has produced a more therapeutic milieu than did the earlier approaches. The feeling of hostility towards the staff which existed in the patient group has largely disappeared. There is a recognition that if a patient has run away that this is a problem for the whole group and does not concern only the nursing staff or the doctor.

Most adolescents with behavior problems use projection as a defense against depression. By holding adults and authority figures responsible for all their misfortunes they manage to avoid any feelings of guilt in spite of their antisocial behavior. In the therapeutic community approach the behavior of each member is examined by the total community, including his peers. The community as a whole gets an insight into the problems of each of its members. The sanctions and any loss of privileges incurred by any member have the approval of the total community. This makes projection as a defense mechanism less effective.

Patients often expressed their concern about a patient who had run away and requested the staff to go with them to bring him back. This sharing of concern and responsibility, which comes from discussing all problems openly as one group and taking part in decision-making processes, has the benefit of not allowing these patients to put the blame for all their frustrations on the staff, as they have done for so long with their parents or other authority figures. They are finally beginning to learn from their mistakes.

Conclusions

Adolescents with behavior problems were found to be unsuitable for treatment in adult wards of the hospital, where the majority of patients suffered from psychotic disorders. The adolescent unit at Douglas Hospital was set up to provide a program specifically designed to meet the needs of these adolescents.

An account has been presented describing the mistakes made and lessons learned in the first 5 years of experiences in the adolescent unit.

On a clinical basis, it appears that the therapeutic community approach is superior to other approaches tried for adolescents with behavior problems.

The hope is that by moving into the field of adolescents with behavior problems it would be possible to up-grade and develop better facilities in the community for this type of patient.

REFERENCES

Adolescent psychiatry (editorial) (1967): Canad. Psychiat. Assoc. J. 97: 1413–1414.

Cameron, K. (1953): Group approach to in-patient adolescents. Amer. J. Psychiat. 109:657–661

Child and Family Clinic (1966): First Annual Report. Douglas Hospital, Montreal.

Hendrickson, W. J., and Holmes, D. J. (1959): Control of behaviour as a crucial factor in intensive psychiatric treatment in an all adolescent ward. Amer. J. Psychiat. 115: 969–973.

Jenkins, R. L. (1962): Diagnosis dynamics and treatment in child psychiatry. In: *Diagnostic Classification of Child Psychiatry; Psychiatric Research Report #18* of the American Psychiatric Association. Washington D. C.

Jenkins, R. L., and Hewitt, L. E. (1944): Types of personality structure encountered in child guidance clinics. Amer. J. Orthopsychiat. 14: 84–94.

Jones, Maxwell (1968): *Beyond the Therapeutic Community: Social Learning and Social Psychiatry.* Yale University Press, New Haven.

Kohlmeyer, W. A., and Rafferty, F. T. (1966): A comprehensive program for adolescents in a state hospital. Curr. Psychiat. Ther. 6: 55–61.

Position statement on psychiatry of adolescence (1967): Amer. J. Psychiat. 123:1031.

Shamsie, S. J.:Evaluating the effectiveness of treatment in an adolescent in-patient unit. To be published.

Shamsie, S. J., and Ellick, E. (1965): Disturbed adolescents, a suggested community approach to treatment. Canad. Psychiat. Assoc. J. 10: 399–404.

Warren, W. (1953): The Adolescent in the Mental Hospital, Medical Press, 230:42–46.

Chapter 10

TREATMENT OF YOUTH IN PRIVATE PRACTICE

Rudolph Wittenberg

THE REFERRAL TRIANGLE

Since adolescents and young adults usually do not make the first contact with the therapist but are referred by a third party, a triangle of interaction is set up which affects the transference. If this constellation can be recognized from the start—the first telephone contact—complications can be avoided during the clinical work.

Often the adolescent patient identifies the referral party with the therapist, particularly since the family or school tends to interpret the function of therapy to the patient. Whenever possible we attempt to structure the interpretation of therapy independently from the referral party. The family, agency, or school which refers the adolescent patient often attempts to be helpful by offering diagnostic clues; at other times a parent may inadvertently announce his hoped-for goals of therapy—all of which has an effect on the adolescent patient and his expectations of therapy. Not infrequently the parent is the one who really asks for help for himself, sending the adolescent patient to be "adjusted" in order to relieve the familial distress. Conflicts in the family sometimes are used to influence the adolescent patient's attitude toward therapy—for or against—depending on the feuding factions in the family.

All of this operates to some degree also with post-adolescent patients, with the additional complication that the role of the referral party is not as overt and directly visible as in adolescence or childhood.

Unlike the adolescent patient, the young adult usually makes his first contact with the therapist directly. But, like the adolescent patient, the post-adolescent too usually does not pay completely for his therapy himself, but has to obtain the consent of family or friends before he can begin treatment. The economic bind, one of the post-adolescent characteristics, influences the patient-therapist relationship from the start. This constellation can affect the transference, quite in the same way as with adolescent patients, unless the therapist insists on a clear separation between his young adult patient and his family, or whatever the source of his financial support. Even when the young adult has nominal control of income—as in cases of inheritance or savings from part-time work—the actual economic dependence is frequently used by the patient as resistance.

Where the end of role-playing (a maturational growth stage, in a patient's major activities of daily life) is combined with the economic bind, it is particularly necessary for the therapist to resist the invasion of family or other referral sources, to avoid being drawn into the referral triangle.

While family or relatives of child or adolescent patients frequently make the first contact with the therapist and attempt to direct the treatment relationship by open suggestions or questions, the referring source in young adult patients usually remains in the background and emerges openly only when the post-adolescent patient asks for interference—usually as part of his resistance or acting-out of negative transference phases.

A young college student who experienced brief states of depersonalization as part of his identity crisis while studying in his parents' home threatened to quit college and work full-time unless the family assisted him with his own apartment. Since this crisis followed an earlier one in which he had lived in a dormitory out of town, as part of the college setup, the family was anxious that he continue in the presently attended second school in his hometown and agreed to pay for his maintenance as long as he would be willing to pay his own rent. The family, which had agreed to the choice of the young adult's therapist, paid for most of the treatment, while the young adult took responsibility for the remainder. When the young adult's acting-out took the form of missing sessions, the family suddenly entered the picture, clearly summoned by the patient. While the therapist had made it clear to patient and family in an early telephone contact that the relationship would have to be strictly confidential and include only the patient and the therapist, the young man had now been using the financial contribution of his family in behalf of his resistance. By letting his family know that he had been missing sessions, he invited them to enter the triangle. The symptoms of oversleeping, coming late for sessions, and missing sessions entirely had been one of his acting-out episodes, which effectively blocked analysis of the transference. In an earlier phase of his analysis he had recognized through several clear dreams that if he could get the therapist to "throw him out" the patient would have considered this a victory in behalf of his moral masochism.

Since the therapist was on guard against this maneuver and had enough insight into his counter-transference not to be challenged by this episode, the patient resorted to a much earlier form of omnipotent acting-out: he again played "mother against father," since he knew that, in his family, mother controlled the money and paid all bills. It was indeed his mother who made contact with the therapist wondering whether she should continue to pay for sessions that were missed since, according to her son, he had not been attending regularly lately. But aside from the waste of money, the mother wondered whether it was good for the son to feel guilty for causing his family expenses that were of no benefit to him.

Clearly, the patient was using the economic bind, the role-playing of earlier childhood, to maneuver therapy into a stalemate. Precisely because he was no longer a young adolescent, but a young adult who paid part of his expenses and lived by himself, the family could not use pressure or heavy authority, but had to leave decisions "up to him."

The opposite situation occurred when a therapist made contact with the family when her patient began to miss sessions and acted-out in other ways. In this case the referral triangle had been more overt from the start, inasmuch as the family, who lived in a distant state from the therapist's office, had made the first contact with the therapist and successfully put her *in loco parentis*. It was as though the therapist had felt responsible to the family, rather than to the brilliant and difficult young undergraduate who was her patient. In addition, the patient came from a wealthy family who had used money to control him and his siblings, doling out the minimum necessary and insisting on exact accounting of all expenses. Of course the family paid all therapeutic expenses, asking for monthly bills, bypassing the patient when it came to discussion of fees, manner of payment, and the entire financial aspect of the therapeutic contract.

By not safeguarding the transference but by acting-out her counter-transference, the therapist lost the patient who said he felt caught in a trap, since the family control which had dominated his entire life now reached into the office of the one person whom he had tried to trust.

Since there was considerable pathologic involvement, the young adult sought and found another therapist who considered that the young man's identity crisis, his self-image dilemma, and the end of role-playing were all so tangled with the economic bind that he (the therapist), after a few preliminary, exploratory sessions and a thorough psychologic diagnostic testing program, arrived at a bold, long-range program: he told the patient that he was very gifted, very mixed up, and that he absolutely needed therapy—but independent of his family, which meant that the patient had to work full-time for a year or two, continue his studies on a part-time basis, and concentrate his energies on working out his problems. Since the young man had not been able to function academically in two of the nation's outstanding colleges, the therapist saw no harm in postponing the patient's academic education for a few years, during which he would experience both the desperately sought-for economic independence from his family's "chains"—as the patient put it—and work intensively on the resolution of his problems, preparing him to function eventually in both school and his profession.

Since the young man was not able to earn enough to pay for his own maintenance and for therapy, the analyst both lowered his fee and made a financial agreement with the patient which would allow him to owe a certain amount until he would be able to repay his debts. This was done on a definite, businesslike basis—comparable to a bank loan— to avoid accumulation of guilt, but based on the patient's personality as the only "security." It was this expression of trust in the sound ego-core of the young adult that formed the foundation of a successful therapeutic relationship. The referral triangle was here bypassed by a definite emphasis on "psychoanalytic treatment as a two-party contractual relationship" (Menninger, 1958).

When the self-image dilemma is particularly severe, the referral triangle poses particular challenges. The daughter of a divorced, successful businesswoman made contact with a therapist "at my mother's suggestion." It became clear in two exploratory interviews that this young college student was caught in her ambivalent strivings, unable to move in any direction without painful conflict against which she had built a defense of smiling indifference and blandness. In spite of the seemingly typical adolescent rebellious attitude toward her mother and authority, the patient was existing in a deeply unconscious symbiotic relationship with her mother, whose control was covered with an attractive liberal and sophisticated veneer.

Because the control was extremely subtle and seemingly reasonable, the young woman had developed a strong, punitive super-ego—in conflict with one of her ego-ideals— which unsuccessfully demanded an equal place in her self-image. Her token rebellions consisted in small, inconsequential feuds with late-room monitors in high school, dormitory supervisors in college, stage managers in the drama lab where she was volunteerng several evenings—over points of order, minor decisions, hairsplitting obsessional details which gave her the illusion of independence. Realistically, because of her inability to invest libido in relationships or work, she was not functioning well in any area and accepted her mother's and college advisor's suggestion that she seek professional help.

The opening sentences of the psychologic report characterize the self image dilemma:

"Although the patient seemed to want to comply with the requirements of the situation, wanted to relate in a pleasant, cooperative manner, underlying negativism and hostility were only thinly veiled. Judging by her test responses, this young woman experiences uncertainty, conflict and at times near-confusion in practically all areas of functioning. No matter what takes place, she does not feel really in tune with what is going on around her or with what she thinks is expected of her, what she should feel or do. . . . "

The young woman felt that she should see a therapist and came with the same pleasant, cooperative manner which the psychologist had noted in her test report, only to display the bland indifference on top of her negativism in every one of her exchanges with the therapist. When the therapist greeted her in the waiting room with a friendly, "good evening," she did not respond except with an enigmatic smile. She made it clear in her particular indirect manner that she was present as a representative of mother and college advisor and would cooperate no matter what.

The patient obediently listed her symptoms—with a few technical terms here and there—and mentioned in passing "even a dream" she had had before coming: "something about walking out of the play in the first act" to which she had some associations which, however, she "did not want to talk about." When the therapist suggested that the patient was not too sure that she needed therapy, the young woman said with a smile that she was not sure about anything and why should she be sure about this? Besides, this was her mother's idea and who knows that it may not do her some good? In the second exploratory interview, the young woman reacted to the therapist with passivity, except to indicate that there had been things on her mind which she, however, did not want to talk about. She was willing to put in an appearance—to appease the super-ego or the incorporated mother image—but unwilling to say things out loud that she could not even admit to herself, in her own mind.

When, in addition, the young woman could not find free hours which coincided with the therapist's schedule, and was unwilling to change her dance class or weekend trips, the therapist suggested that the patient might wait with therapy until later in her life, when she felt that this was necessary. He shared some of the psychologic findings, outlined the broad area of her ambivalence, and invited her to return when her schedule would coincide with his. He supported her ego-ideal by emphasizing the casually mentioned wish to have her own apartment, as a very understandable idea, and hoped that she would be able to carry out this plan before too long.

The therapist further safeguarded the potential relationship by not sharing anything with the mother who called to inquire why her daughter was not receiving treatment and by a tactful explanation of why an interview with the mother would not be wise.

When, a year later, a crisis developed in the young woman's relationship with her boyfriend—which she in part blamed on the lack of privacy—the defense of indifference and blandness began to crumble enough to bring the self-image dilemma to a head. At this point, the patient wrote a note to the therapist, inquiring whether he "cared to see me" and began therapy.

She started her first session with the ego-ideal support from the exploratory interview 12 months earlier: the search for a home of her own.

It would seem as though in this situation, where the self-image dilemma had been particularly severe, the referral triangle posed a temporary impasse to therapy, as long as the super-ego representative—the energetic mother —determined the motivation for therapy. Both the expressed confidence in the patient's wishes to wait with treatment—though not openly verbalized—and the support of her wish for her own apartment represented a strengthening of the ego-ideal, which, after an acute crisis in her life, tipped the balance of the dilemma enough for the patient to consider resolving the ambivalent strivings.

In this and the previous illustrations of the referral triangle, the family of the patient represented one of the three sides. There are many, equally complex situations in which the referral of a young adult has not come from the family—directly or indirectly—but originated with a member of the community. In these instances also we need to be alert to the potential of a referral triangle with the ensuing complications for therapy. The following illustration may clarify this further.

A young graduate student was referred by a neighbor, a high-school teacher who had some previous professional contact with the therapist. It was not the patient himself who made the first contact but the teacher, who had come to know the patient through the patient's relationships with her daughter.

The teacher had become concerned about the young man's anxiety, his loss of weight, and what she considered a paranoid trend, which she believed the young man may have "taken over from his mother" who had been in a state hospital for several years with a diagnosis of "paranoid schizophrenia." Since the young man was not only her daughter's boyfriend but had also become somebody the teacher herself was very fond of, she was very concerned that he work out his problems.

The teacher had "taken the liberty of suggesting professional help for him" and had mentioned the therapist's name. The young man—she reported—had asked her to make the first contact.

The young therapist, who was not particularly concerned about the danger of a referral triangle, gave the woman an appointment for the patient and, with this simple step, set in motion the complications of a triangular relationship, with all the classical oedipal features. Because of a mistaken sense of professional courtesy—or perhaps because he needed the good will of a potential referral source for the future—the therapist failed to separate the referral source from the patient by not asking the young man to call himself for an appointment. He allowed the teacher to make the appointment and agreed to her suggestion to keep the fee as modest as possible because of the young man's strained circumstances.

When the young man arrived for his first session, he behaved exactly as an adolescent who had been sent by his mother, using the referral source to enforce his resistances: "Mrs. Frey suggested that I see you."

This familiar gambit can be avoided if we ask potential adolescent patients to call for their first appointment. It is certainly a requirement for young adults.

While this initial delay can be overcome in a relatively short time, the involvement of the referral party in the treatment process is more complicated.

For the first 2 years of his therapy, the patient used the teacher who had referred him to reenact the childhood pattern of playing mother against father. When he could not accept the fee set by the therapist, when he could not accept an interpretation, and when he repressed hostile feelings in the transference, he poured them out to his neighbor, the teacher-mother-referral party. The teacher, in turn, having been responsible for the therapeutic contact, took it upon herself to side with or against the patient, to attempt to influence the therapist by telephone or letters, and on two occasions asked for an appointment.

The therapist allowed this interference by continuing occasional contacts with the teacher, although her interference never came through associations by the patient. Indeed, the patient censored his contacts with the teacher, particularly remarks that were critical of the therapist. When once, after a particularly long pause, the therapist inquired into the silence, the patient blushed and explained that he had just run into the teacher on the street who wanted to know how much longer therapy would last. Since this had been the first comment about the referral source, the therapist encouraged his patient to tell him more about these inquiries and suggested that the patient may have mixed feelings about a neighbor wanting to know so much about his therapy. It was then that the patient expressed his first hostile feelings about the "nosy" neighbor to whom he probably should be very grateful but toward whom he also felt resentful. Since this young man had had real difficulties facing his homosexual conflicts, the long delay in associating freely had unnecessarily complicated the complex transference. Much of this could have been bypassed if the therapist had been aware of the many ways which the referral triangle can lead to acting-out of the oedipal situation in post-adolescence.

THE OPENING PHASE

In order to create from the beginning a climate in which the watchfulness of the super-ego can be relaxed, we want to avoid comments or attitudes that suggest watchfulness on our part, i.e., we do not want to create the impression that the post-adolescent patient is being watched or judged in any way. In practical terms we would avoid "shrewd or insightful" observations or any suggestions that sound like special insights or an awareness of the patient's problems that he himself has not already expressed.

After the therapeutic process has been under way for a time, during which we attempt to modify the severities of his rigid super-ego structures, our young adult patient will use us most likely as his super-ego to avoid increase of guilt or as a protection against acting-out. However, this development cannot start in the beginning and in no case during the consultation, in which this climate may easily lead to negative transference, unnecessarily complicating the work ahead.

As it is, we will have to demand a certain fee, announce certain hours which may complicate the patient's life and introduce some basic rules—in short, we are, *nolens volens,* in a somewhat authoritarian position, in addition to the awe in which many young people hold workers in our profession. When Glover cautions against "too spurious a professional attitude" and states that "the besetting sins of psycho-analytical practice are smugness, timidity, hypersensitivity and ritualism" (Glover, 1955A), we would suggest that this is particulary valid for the young adult who, because of his position, is himself hypersensitive to any behavior that smacks of parental authority.

On the other side, young adults have complained about the false joviality and condescending neutrality which they have encountered in initial consultations. In order not to structure the transference, some therapists begin their passive listening as soon as possible after the young adult has entered the office, creating unnecessary tension and anxiety in the patient who cannot know what is expected of him.

We do structure the transference, whether we are active or passive, and for this reason it would seem advisable to be definite in the image we are creating from tha start. The more we succeed in remaining on the level that the patient has reached, the more the patient can accept our demands. For a simple illustration, take the matter of how to address the patient on first sight in the waiting room. It seems natural and realistic to address him by the name which he himself has used in his first telephone contact with us: "You are Bob Jones, I am Dr. Smith." This would be different from introducing ourselves to a young adolescent who has been referred as "Bob" and would feel alienated if we did not say, "Hi, Bob." Young adults are sensitive about being addressed by a stranger by their first name only, but would feel awkward if we used the conventional "Mr." If the referral has been made by a third party, it is helpful to ask what the young adult patient calls himself.

If we are not sure how to address the patient, we might ask him and get a first glimpse at the self-image dilemma. A young graduate student explained that his name was "Robert Hartley the Second, after my father and graddfather. My parents call me Bob, but I prefer just plain 'Chuck.'" When interest was expressed in the origin of this nickname, he said that this was his fraternity name, and began to talk about the significance of his reference group, his girlfriend, and led into his conflict over his self-image dilemma. We had, in fact, begun our diagnostic interview.

In this opening phase we also establish the basic tone between therapist and patient. In spite of the mature veneer of many post-adolescent patients and their often outstanding intellectual maturity, the young adults seem to require some of the same active, outgoing attitude on our part that we have come to develop with adolescents. If we use the concept of compassionate neutrality as a basic analytic attitude with all our patients, the accent might well be on "compassionate" when it comes to young adults, who have come for resolution of basic conflicts and feel particularly ambivalent toward the process from the start, in part as a result of the self-image dilemma.

In addition to the expected resistance—the basic omnipotent position—which we will have to work with throughout the analytic process, there is another form of realistic interference which is in large measure due to the characteristics of the post-adolescent situation. Many young adults who have come to the conclusion that they need professional help have usually read a good deal, taken courses in various aspects of pscyhology, and discussed forms of psychotherapy or schools of analytic thought. This intellectual interest often leaves them quite troubled and confused, doubtful over what they should expect and suspicious of what they hear from teachers, older friends, or the therapist whom they came to see.

It is a truism to state that this intellectual hesitation and doubt will be used in the service of the unconscious resistances; however, we cannot help but deal first with the surface interferences if we hope to get a chance to reach the basic ones. Contrary to the maneuvers of adolescent patients and quite different from the manifest rationalizations of adult patients, early resistances of post-adolescent patients cannot be countered by a withdrawal to a passive position, which will be experienced as an evasion of their questions. If young adults ask about analytic orientation, our theoretic position, or schools of training, we would gain in the long run if we attempted to answer their often misplaced and confusing questions as directly and simply as we are able to. While it is axiomatic, as Glover suggests, that "nothing is more obstructive to analytic progress than to commence work by taking sides on controversial issues," we also cannot afford to evade young adults' rationalizations by withdrawal to humorless or stodgy pronouncements about our professional role.

Questions sometimes arise in connection with patients' concern over the use of the couch. Since analysis is considered the "real thing" and since the cliché associates the process with the use of the couch, many young adults have questions about it.

Inasmuch as we are here considering not a complete, classical analysis but a more limited analytic therapy, the question arises whether the use of a couch is altogether appropriate. In spite of the many different practices currently in vogue, there is probably agreement that the couch should not be used with severely regressed or some borderline patients, who cannot make the transition from free association to reality, from primary- to secondary-process thinking without impairing their daily functioning. Sometimes younger therapists have suggested the use of the couch without being fully aware of the main function of this position: to encourage the development of a transference neurosis, as part of the classical analysis. While the use of the couch for other purposes may or may not be harmful to the therapeutic process, it would certainly not be helpful to ask a post-adolescent patient to use the couch in order to encourage his illusion that he is "under analysis"—getting the most intensive therapy possible. As a general practice with young adults, sitting up during a twice-a-week appointment has been satisfactory. There are exceptions, of course, particularly when it has become obvious that the associations are severely restricted by sitting up and facing the therapist. However, we might be wary when young adults ask about the couch in the beginning, and first explore what this inquiry represents.

Aside from the possible use of the couch as an acting-out of resistance, the sitting up in twice-a-week analytic therapy may be considered a safeguard, particularly with adolescents in whom the differentiation between age-specific characteristics and genuine borderline states is not easy to make, at least in the opening phase of treatment.

At the same time, just because we are trying to create

an informal atmosphere, we want to be sure to watch for the many familiar forms of resistances. Among these are: starting the session in the waiting room or bringing up important material or dreams at the end of the hour or on the way out (in other words, avoiding the structure of the analytic relationship by turning it into a social discussion session), making frequent phone calls to the analyst, canceling appointments, making changes in appointments frequently, bringing a friend to the waiting room while the session is in progress, avoiding discussion of payments, paying the monthly bill at irregular intervals or forgetting to pay, delaying the session by making out the check in the office, and receiving phone calls in the analyst's office. These are some of the characteristic resistances, particularly noted in the beginning of the therapeutic relationship. It has often been helpful, particularly with young adults in college, to state the ground rules in the beginning of the relationship. Many post-adolescent patients have been conditioned to expect some statement of procedures and rules. One young adult put it well when he said to his therapist, after having accepted the need for treatment, "How do we go about it?"

Particularly with the bright and sophisticated young adult, it is helpful to be very candid about the whole of the therapeutic process: the difficulties in learning to free-associate, the probable length of therapy, the possible results one can reasonably expect. Intelligent young people are offended when they are told to just go ahead and say whatever comes to mind, as though this were an easy task; they feel talked down to when somebody tells them that the length of treatment "depends"; they rightfully feel treated as children when they ask about the results of therapy and are told that they have to "wait and see." They feel that these answers are not sincere, but evasive generalizations, designed to establish the oracle-like wisdom of the therapist. The responses are never intended as an expression of modesty or lack of knowledge on our part, although either may in reality account for them.

The bright, young adult who has relied on his intellect to cope with his ego deficiencies will need considerable encouragement to allow himself to express thoughts and feelings that "make no sense" at the moment, that seem illogical or irrational. It may be helpful to anticipate this difficulty and let him know that everything within him and his previous training will object to letting out "meaningless" or "ridiculous" sentences or ideas. We might be more helpful and realistic to point out in the beginning that it will take time to learn this new way of speaking.

When young people have been realistically concerned with the usual length of the therapeutic experience, I have sometimes found it helpful to refer to such statistics as the length of training of analytic students in the major training institutes in the United States as reported by Lewin and Ross (1960) who found that 800 hours were the average time required for a full analysis, with allowance for variations. Since we frequently do not plan a full analysis, it seems realistic to refer to this figure as a general guideline and to emphasize that although, in the work planned, less time will be required, it will take a few hundred hours in any case to produce any significant changes. The young adult, used to thinking in terms of years of collge or graduate school, does not usually realize that 2 hours of weekly therapy add up to about 100 hours a year, with vacations. It is realistic to ask them to plan for staying two or three years at least, if the work and money invested are to be worth the effort. That this means planning their study or work, their residence and budget is understood.

Contrary to the views of some colleagues, I cannot find the young adult's question about the results of analytic therapy unjustified. He has a right to ask what he can expect for the work and money invested, just as with any other service rendered in our society. Indeed, if one cannot anticipate the modification of some very troublesome symptoms, the reduction of pain that interferes with the pleasure of living, the resolution of some of the major interferences, a clarification of the self-image dilemma, and a more realistic approach to the problems of everyday life, one might do better to refer the prospective patient to somebody else. Certainly we can give no written guarantees, but we can make reasonable assumptions, based on our professional experience and confidence. We anticipate hard work on the part of ourselves and our patient, but unless we can have a positive expectation for the outcome it will be very difficult for the patient to sustain the many dark moments in the therapeutic process.

STYLES OF FREE ASSOCIATION

The language of our patient is always of diagnostic interest because the change in the manner of expression, rhetoric and rhythm of speech, and variance in choice of certain words or repetition of others reflect varying ego states, and often are the first indicators of thinking disorders.

That patients ask for reassurance in their chain of associations is expected. How they ask for it should be distinguished. A patient may ask, "Do I make myself clear?" or he may ask, "Does this sound reasonable?" or he may, after several attempts to express a feeling add, "Did you get what I mean?" That obsessive patients take great pains in trying to find the right word is axiomatic; what words they reject or accept is of interest. Style of speech may change during an analysis as dream content does: use of concrete or abstract words; appropriateness of metaphors; use of symbolic language.

With the post-adolescent patient we may obtain meaningful leads into the particular post-adolescent characteristics in addition to the manifest and latent content by paying particular attention to his style of free association.

Certain *depersonalization* states as representative of identity diffusion can frequently be seen in young adults who not only have difficulty in beginning a sentence but whose ego fragmentation leads to trailing off toward the end of a statement, to the extent that they usually do not finish a sentence. Their speech resembles a heavily revised or edited manuscript, in which words are crossed out, replaced, written over, circled and inserted above or below the lines. Their voice may be low in volume and their speech accompanied by inappropriate hand movements which bear no relevance to the content of the communication. They, of course, have been told about their manner of speaking by family, school, or friends and know the effect of their speech pattern, so that its use in therapy can be considered another tool in behalf of their resistances; however, the particular form it had taken over a period of years is of interest. It would seem that the language, speech, and voice pattern may be studied by itself, instead of looking at it in a generalized way as a "resistance."

There will be variations in the speech pattern and degrees of unfinished or inaudible associations. Contrary to expectation, there does not seem to be any surface connection between the pattern and the content: the speech pattern is not directly related to a particularly embarrassing or difficult association. We probably should consider the pattern as a symptom and observe it the way we do any symptom—as a barometer of degrees of ego integration.

The pattern presents certain clinical problems since the unconscious purpose is, in fact, accomplished: often what the patient is saying is not understood by the therapist. In the beginning, when they have not yet understood this symptom sufficiently, some therapists will tell the patient that they had not been able to hear what he had been saying. They are, in fact, asking the patient to speak up. This kind of intervention may be used in behalf of the resistance (the patient feels that he was successful with his broken speech) or it may be used for acting-out of the transference authority (the patient will apologize and for a few moments speak up and force himself to complete a sentence). A more clinically useful response would be to treat this kind of depersonalized speech as a fragment, similar to a dream fragment or a partial memory, that is, to identify with the patient and mentally fill in what he had not been able to complete with articulate words. This response is not possible for every clinician or at all times, since the broken speech is often interpreted as hostility and reacted to with some degree of irritation.

The sophisticated young adult who has read about "free association" and comes to us with a set expectation of his behavior may cope with the depersonalization of speech by a number of reaction formations against the unacceptable broken-up sentence. One of the most common devices is the word-bridge, a frequent insertion of the word "and" between ends of half-sentences to give himself and us the impression that he is indeed "associating." The word-bridge is pronounced in a slow and drawn-out manner, to give himself time for a new thought or expression of feeling. While it is true that this is related to isolation—one of the common defenses—it is of interest also in the above-mentioned connection.

Another way in which young people tend to cope with the broken-speech pattern is the run-on speech, comparable to run-on sentences, without commas, semicolons, or periods. Their pattern of association resembles an unbroken page of print, without paragraphs or interruptions. This method of flooding the therapist with words may or may not represent a reaction against the broken-speech pattern, but one may find a return to the unfinished sentence once one intervenes into the run-on speech.

Most typically, the voice and affect are flat in the monotone flooding—again, not directly related to the content of the material.

A very different style of speech may be observed when the adolescent struggles with the *end of role-playing* and demonstrates the variety of roles that he had been enacting in different language patterns. It would not be unusual to find quite different modes of speech in one session. The young adult may, for example, act out the role of the detached "intellectual" by interlacing every association with terms borrowed from his psychology classes or from popular reading on psychoanalysis. He will not say "mixed up" but "ambivalent"; instead of saying "angry" he will "feel hostile"; instead of telling us that he "forgot a dream," he will say that he "repressed it." When a therapist comments on this defense, the patient may give it up and instead shift to the use of more weighty words in the description of everyday events. He will not have "bought" a magazine, but "purchased" it; instead of "thinking of" changing a course, he is "considering the possibility."

The same patient may, in the same hour, shift gears to the role of the member of his reference group and talk in "hip" language, which represents another role he has been playing and is considering giving up. If the therapist comments on the changed speech pattern the patient will feel that he has been "put down" in addition to all the "bread" he is paying for this "scene." While he may have commented earlier on the complicated break-up with his girl friend in perhaps oversophisticated terms, he will now refer to this by saying that "Jane and I split"—two different roles, expressed in different languages, representing the ease with which he can shift from one to the other or, we may say, suggesting that he is not deeply involved in either role.

As for choices of clinical intervention, it would seems that the role diffusion would take precedence over deeper, instinctual conflicts. In terms of the young adult mentioned above, we would first try to understand the need for the shift in language before we could penetrate to the unconscious causes of his "splitting" with his girl friend, particularly since brief, intensive relationships had been a pattern with this patient. The change in style of his free association may give us the opportunity to observe a form of acting-out of role-playing, which we had earlier referred to as a more primitive mode of attempted problem-solving. The language may be viewed as a form of externalization—as in all acting-out—or as an attempt to extend the role-playing beyond its time. To the degree to which the post-adolescent has come to an end of role-playing, the language shifts represent a transference resistance which requires interpretation.

The *self-image* is frequently made more transparent by the predominance of the super-ego or the ego-ideal in the young adult patient, as illustrated by the following:

> The patient, a young man who on occasion had difficulty in pronouncing words, regressed to a stammering pattern which had characterized a brief period prior to the beginning of adolescence. Although he had completely overcome this handicap, traces of it would occur either during some sessions or for a few consecutive hours during a week. This seemed at first related to aim-inhibited expressions, directly related to the latent content of the material. On further observation, however, it became clearer that the speech pattern was determined by the interference of the severe super-ego, while there was no difficulty in associating freely when the ego-ideal aspect of the self-image was predominant. It was of interest to note that when the super-ego was too predominant, the patient not only had difficulty in speaking but there was also a difference in the choice of words. While he would usually speak in a light vein, using

casual words and some humor, the language would become ponderous and heavy, the voice would tighten, and the flow slow down to a near halt in speech.

At such times the patient would not report dreams freely from memory, but would refer to a piece of paper on which he had noted them down upon awakening. There would then be few associations following the written report of the dream; instead, there were long silences, with references to the piece of paper. On the other hand, when the ego-ideal aspect of the self-image was predominant, the patient's memory was much less restricted, and dreams and associations came easily and creatively, with no concern with order or logic.

The difference in the speech pattern can be better understood if one recalls that speech originally is set in motion, like any other organ function, "through aim-inhibited sexual strivings, desexualized libido and thus is the expression of sublimation which begins very early" (Nunberg, 1955).

Nunberg suggests in the same context that if the speech-forming ego becomes flooded with libido, in other words, if the cerebral cortex or the speech apparatus (larynx, mouth), or both at the same time, becomes eroticized, a disturbance of the function of speech is the result. This disturbance is expressed in a regression of the ego, in relation to speech, to its magical phase of operation.

In the post-adolescent phase of development, in which the crisis of the self-image may be viewed as a conflict between super-ego and differing ego-ideals, the disturbance of the function of speech is frequently represented in a stalemate, expressed in periods of silence. If the therapist should attempt to help the patient with this mode of silent communication by inquiring "what comes to mind," it is likely that he will get no reply, because the young adult is caught in the self-image predicament or, in instinctual terms, the ego is too dammed up with libido to allow any free flow of speech. The chance for overcoming this handicap is better if the clinician addresses himself either to the ego-ideal ("you feel it best to cool it now?") or the super-ego ("shouldn't we see what is interfering now?") aspects of the patient's ego rather than to the total self, which at this moment is in a crisis. The open-ended question is likely to produce more anxiety or withdrawal at this point.

Another aspect of late adolescence which is often expressed in the style of free association is the *cognition of time continuity*. As with the alternation of speech behavior, observable in the end of role-playing and the self-image quandary, this characteristic also is visible in two contrasting manners of talking. After the cognition of time continuity had been repressed or denied for a period, this is then followed by a sharp awareness of the reality of time having passed, leading to a sudden anxiety in the speech pattern. The young adult quite suddenly finds himself flooded with a panic-like state which demands that he leave no moment unused in the session, but that he talk without interruption. He experiences the hour as a 50-minute void which he must fill with his associations, speaking rapidly and, as one young adult expressed it, "as if you are a sports announcer on the radio waiting for the athletes to appear in the ring and having to fill in empty time continuously." He may comment on his manner of speaking by suggesting, with some sarcasm, that he must not waste a minute, that time keeps on moving and every moment counts. One young adult used the Latin *"carpe diem"* and the attendant philosophy to explain his anxiety.

This may be followed by periods of near-lethargic speech or long drawn-out interruptions and pauses, which are explained by the fact that there is plenty of time, that after all time is meaningless by itself or, as one witty student put it, time matters little "in the infinite scheme of things."

It is of interest to note that this vascillating attitude toward time, expressed in the style of speaking, seems to go parallel with the patient's use of time during the day or night. It ranges from a minimum of work to a very tight schedule in which every moment seems to count.

The clinical problem lies in the necessity of making a choice between accepting the particular language of many post-adolescent patients or inquiring into some of the concepts, which frequently are short-cut expressions, as part of the style of speech belonging to one of the reference groups. The young adult, for example, who has identified with some of the currently popular "hip" groups and as part of this identification has adopted their language, assumes that we know that he means "money" when he speaks of "bread." While there is no clinical problem in learning the typical language of each patient, there is a problem when it comes to more than slang or occasional words, such as complex concepts expressed in shorthand abbreviations.

The young adult patient will tell us that her friend "turned her off," or she might say that he is "dragging her." These are two fairly typical expressions which are graphic and pert and can be understood in social conversation. However, as part of an association, we may have to understand more than the fact that the friend "turned her off." Is she repelled by him quite suddenly or as part of a development of their relationship; is she referring to a mood of an hour or a night; is she reacting to an impulse, to aspects of his character that she had not experienced before? In other words, we are dealing with the familiar problem of when to inquire into the patient's association, whether to ask for elaboration or choose instead to let the associations flow without our interruption. This is, of course, a basic problem of interpretation which we shall discuss later. However, in some adolescent patients, this is complicated by the consideration of the patient's language.

Do we use the patient's language for our inquiry: "What turned you off?" or do we rephrase it in more conventional language? The latter would require something resembling translation from a foreign language, including the difficulties inherent in rendering a word in different tongues. Should we say: "What upset you?" or "What repelled you suddenly?" Neither may represent the meaning of the words "turning off."

For another typical illustration, take a concept like "he dragged me." It can be understood to mean: "depressed me," "bored me," or, as one patient explained, "made me feel like nothing." In other words, we don't precisely know what the patient is saying, what feeling is being conveyed by this short-cut expression.

In using his slang for our inquiry, the young adult patient may feel that we are trespassing or "putting him down"; in rephrasing the lingo in conventional language, we may appear stuffy or "square." This is one dilemma. That we inquire at all—whether in slang or nonslang— may well be used in behalf of the resistance by the patient in reacting to our lack of understanding of the language, rather than in us determining the underlying meaning. Not to inquire at all may be considered as a sign of lack of interest on our part, since the sophisticated young adult is well aware of the fact that his language—like his long hair or dress—is meant to emphasize the difference between his group, his tradition, and the conventional world around him. Like the orthodox Jew, the anti-establishment young adult intends to emphasize his difference by a markedly different appearance and language. Young people look for reactions of surprise, indignation, envy, contempt—any number of reactions except indifference. If we do not inquire into his language, do not react for clinical reasons, he will often feel that we are, in fact, hostile through our silence. While this is a common transference reaction in analytic patients, it takes on another dimension when the language by itself would call for comment, aside from the meaning of the communication.

The silence of the patient, too, takes on another dimension with those young adults whose reference groups emphasize detachment, lack of reaction, and a minimum of communication. When we tend to think of long silences as representing resistances in our patients, we probably should consider, in some young adult patients, that, by their standards of "cool" behavior, silence is the preferred form of "communication," as one young adult put it, citing as his authority the composer Cage, who wrote and performed compositions which consist of silence, or some avant-garde painters whose canvases consist of blank white spaces, described as "white on white."

No matter what the clinician's attitude toward the expressions of the current culture of young adults may be, these expressions will have to be understood as part of the cultural background against which our young adult patients grew up. We could almost think of this milieu as an alien culture, almost comparable to a Japanese woman patient who would talk to us with greater ease if she knew that we understood her culture, in which the woman is expected to walk—literally and symbolically—behind the man. We are used to adaptations to patients from foreign cultures, while we usually do not think of our young adult patients, born and raised in our country, as aliens. For some of them, the cultural differences almost amount to the same as those of patients of different cultures. Their culture will determine their way of speaking and make for a different style of free association from that which we are used to in contacts with our contemporary patients.

Just because we are concerned with safeguarding the classical content of analytic work, it is necessary to be particularly alert to the many ways in which the young adult reveals his complex personality in his communication with us. The matter of our reaction to this style of association will depend in part on our intuitive grasp of these patient's messages, in part on our ability to handle them with tact and sensitivity.

ON INTERVENTION AND INTERPRETATION

The essential difference between variation and modification of analytic technique, between exploration and education, is the reliance on interpretation instead of manipulative intervention, on insight achieved through verbalization and working though, in favor of transference results or so-called corrective emotional experiences. Applied to the characteristics of adolescent patients, with whom a full analytic experience is not always possible, this would mean a variation in the style of interpretations, without over-reliance on intellectualizations and suggestions.

To sharpen up this style of interpretation we should recall that, even in the classical analysis, suggestions are used, which we label interventions (questions re: duration of a symptom; re: connection to the past). The difference between suggestions in analytic therapy and in educational manipulation seem to be this:

In a classical analysis, suggestions are used as steps that eventually lead up to an interpretation; in the educational kind of therapy, suggestions are used per se, as substitutes for interpretations. In the former, transference is used as a transmission belt that makes re-experiencing possible; in the latter, transference is used as a substitute for the original authority figures: we become the better parent, more objective, more loving, but still with the authority of "knowing better." Hence we speak in educational therapy of transference authority or transference results.

In the more limited form of analytic therapy, we would not use any more leading-up suggestions than in a full analytic experience. The difference would lie in the "depth" of interpretation.

The question of definition of "depth of interpretation" has been raised many times and probably not fully answered. However, previous discussions have helped us to become more aware of the complexity of the concept. As the research questionnaire reported by Glover (1955B) suggests, the concept of depth has been defined both in terms of degree of repression and inaccessibility to consciousness. The term has been used to connote either developmental levels or degrees of repression, and there seems to be agreement on the idea that "deep is a word that belongs in the first instance to the sphere of 'topographic' description."

Altogether, the concept of depth suggests the older ideas of the Unconscious existing below the level of the Preconscious and the Conscious, as expressed by Freud in his classical iceberg metaphoric concept.

The shift from the topographic to the structural theory not only has given needed emphasis to maturation and developmental phases (such as post-adolescence), but it also has definite bearing on our therapeutic task, in particular our mode of interpretation. While in the topographic theory the purpose of interpretations had been to make the unconscious conscious, in the structural theory "conflicts over moral demands are accounted for in terms of the super-ego . . . it is important to make the patient conscious not only of the instinctual aspects of his conflicts but of their defensive and super-ego aspects as well, with careful attention to the content of anxieties involved" (Greenacre, 1952).

It is the super-ego aspect of the conflicts of our adolescent patients that will be interpreted differently from those of our adult patients, because of the characteristics of this phase of growth.

The super-ego aspect of the neurotic conflicts of our

adolescent patients will require a less decisive interpretation than of our adult patients for two distinct reasons. First, because of the recognition that, for example, in regression we now recognize the temporary nature of both drive and ego regression, we are not as impressed with the "depth" of the regression as with the effect it may have on adaptation. Second, the super-ego aspects of the conflicts cannot be as sharply isolated for an interpretation, because in adolescence it is not always possible to distinguish between super-ego and ego-ideal, so that we cannot be as definitive in our interpretations as we might be with patients whose self-image dilemma is less acute. This is further confirmed by Arlow and Brenner, who, in discussing regression, suggest that "transient ego regressions may be observed in both normal and pathological contexts. They form the basis of such phenomena as temporary disturbances in the sense of *identity,* transient episodes of *depersonalization* . . . and disturbances in the sense of *time* . . . " (Arlow and Brenner, 1964)—all characteristics of adolescence! It is axiomatic that such regressions occur in analytic therapy with many patients, while they still form a nucleus of what may be called a normal state of adolescence.

It would follow that with adolescent patients—with less well-established ego boundaries, the self-image dilemma, identity symptoms, end of role-playing, and time confusion—our interpretations would have to be more tentative than with adult patients. To some degree we have to be as aware of the fluidity of ego states as with borderline cases, although there will be periods in which we seem to have achieved more stability of the boundaries and seem to be dealing with a sound ego core.

This is another special aspect of interpretations in adolescent patients. Unlike the adult patient with a well-developed neurotic core, with the young adult patient we do not always know what we are dealing with.

When we have degrees of a pathologic condition in all the areas that constitute adolescence, it is sometimes difficult to determine which area requires interpretation first. The following is presented as an example.

A young graduate student, who had worked so brilliantly but erratically that he had been asked to drop out of the program of one of our most prominent universities, brought little material on his serious work interferences, but felt obsessively compelled to report his acute conflicts with two of his girl friends, while his lack of recogintion of time continuity prevented him from being on time for his sessions or for class—indeed, prevented him frequently from waking up in time for a 10 o'clock morning session.

To get this patient to consider this aspect of his super-ego, ego-ideal conflict was difficult because it was not ego-syntonic and remained uncathected, in spite of the fact that he had to recognize the unreality of his frequently missed sessions. This recognition, however, was distorted by his identification with his current reference group in which "time" was considered as another pressure by the establishment to codify and organize life. To be free, according to this group, one did neither wear a watch, nor ever bother thinking of time, hours or days, but one remained concentrated on the inner "creative" self. It was, of course, understandable that this young man had a particularly rigid and successful father who was as precise with time as he was with money or verbal expressions. It is also significant, as an illustration of the economic bind, that this father at first refused to pay for his son's therapy because the choice of the analyst had been the young man's instead of the father's. The young adult, who had seen several therapists chosen by his father, determined to remain with the therapist of his choice, and, instead of engaging in a futile battle with his father, asked for the cash value of his educational policy which was due at this time. He was now able to pay for his treatment, but considered the money his father's nevertheless. With this gambit he could further rationalize that the money wasted for missed sessions was not really his.

Clearly, for practical reasons, the matter of missed sessions, and sessions lasting 20 minutes had to be faced if the patient were to benefit from treatment. At the same time, interpretations that would make the therapist sound like father would obviously not be indicated. To strengthen the pseudo-ego-ideal by ignoring the issue would not help the ego to develop sounder boundaries leading toward more realistic adaptation.

It appears that the transference became part of the post-adolescent self-image crisis, requiring first a series of suggestions that would eventually lead to an interpretation which the patient's ego could tolerate.

With an adult patient who is firmly committed to a profession or a line of work that provides the means of paying for therapy, one might choose not to intervene in the super-ego conflict, expressed in frequently missed sessions, until the patient is ready to bring it up.

In the case of the young graduate student, the interpretation aimed at the super-ego conflict was prepared by a number of progressive suggestions, beginning with nothing more than a tilted head—a silent questioning of his routine apology for being late again. In subsequent sessions, when the patient repeated his "sorry I'm late" cliché, the therapist by not reassuring him in the cliché manner led the young adult to the point where he himself noticed that he was being repetitious in both the fact of being quite late and sliding over it with the same phrase. Here the therapist nodded agreement, together with an accepting smile that encouraged the patient to dwell on the symptom a little longer than before.

For the first time the patient experienced and began to face up to the fact that there were forces inside his mind over which he had no control: he had reported how he had set two alarm clocks, used a telephone waking service, and put the clocks far away from his bed—all this after having gone to bed at a reasonable hour. In spite of his considerable intellectual knowledge of unconscious processes, this was the first time that he *"recognized"* the existence of the unconscious, of forces from the past which made him do things that he rationally had not willed.

At this point a careful interpretation aimed at the ego regression could be made, without involving the labile super-ego state, without aggravating the super-ego, ego-ideal dilemma, and without complicating the transference.

By interpreting the ego regression as a step backward to earlier stages of gratification, the super-ego guilt was neutralized or even reduced.

"Educational" suggestions, such as, "Something inside you didn't want to come here," would have bypassed the ego regression, activated the super-ego conflict, increased guilt, and complicated the transference and countertransference.

That the ego-regression interpretation was of some therapeutic value was evidenced by the release of early memories: playing on the railroad tracks at 4 years of age without hearing the train and being rescued by an older sister: jumping out of the family car before it had come to a complete stop—new material on impaired adaptation and reality testing as resulting from earlier ego fractures. The obvious masochistic component of the character structure was not highlighted at this point, since the patient was just now beginning to make contact with the concept of partial ego regression and its effect on his present-day life.

The shift from present to past to present, and the relative emphasis form another aspect of special interest in the interpretation of material when dealing with young adults. Because of the characteristics of this phase of growth, present-day manifestations or behavior will be avoided by the patient, while repeating already conscious memories that he is experiencing as less painful. Since the patient can use the rationalization that in analysis one tries to remember, he feels at peace with his super-ego, while in reality the most difficult aspect of the analytic process is being avoided. The young adult, to whom we referred above, found it much more comfortable to dwell on the early memories—even discovering new ones—than to cope with the present-day difficulty of coming on time for his analysis or his classes in school.

Such a situation presents something of a dilemma for the clinician, who is inclined to regard recovery of forgotten memories as of greater therapeutic yield than the temporary, although necessary, modification of current symptoms which interfere with daily living. Probably with this more limited form of analytic therapy—both with adults and adolescents—some more time will have to be given to the ability to cope in the present with such elementary tasks as arriving for the therapeutic hour in reasonable time or attending classes in graduate school with a modicum of regularity. To accomplish this, without damaging the positive transference and without stirring up super-ego conflicts, is a particular challenge, especially in the opening phase of analytic therapy. Also, we do not want to create the impression that we are less interested in early memories and analysis of dreams than in the more mundane, practical daily chores of living.

Probably the guiding line will be the patient's ability to tolerate some of the anxiety that accompanies insights.

Greenacre (1952), Schur (1953) and Zetzel (1949 and 1953) have emphasized the connection between a patient's ability to bear anxiety and psychologic insight. Zetzel suggests that "limitations, inherent in the earlier developmental failure . . . influence the degree to which persons predisposed to great anxiety can respond successfully to traditional psychoanalytical technique . . . in the analysis of neurotic patients this capacity (to recognize and tolerate the existence of an internal, unconsciously determined danger situation) of achieving and tolerating the anxiety associated with insight is of decisive importance . . . " (Zetzel, 1949 and 1953).

This highlights the topic of anxiety in analysis and in analytic therapy, and raises the technical problem of *reassurance* as an intervention or one of the suggestive steps leading up to an interpretation. While there is agreement on the danger of rigidity in such modifying devices as reassurance, either for or against, the attitudes of analysts differ widely, depending on their theoretic positions. As with the management of super-ego conflicts in adolescence, the matter of reassurance too cannot be left to chance in the hope that transference authority can accomplish what in the long run requires slow uncovering and interpretation.

Schmideberg commented on this particular aspect in an earlier paper, when she suggested that "the fact that pseudo-analysts use reassurance instead of interpretation, or use it in a wrong way, should not prevent one from using it correctly, that is, combined with interpretation." She compared reassurance in analysis to narcosis in surgery, and most classical analysts seemed to be of the opinion that "while it might be a useful adjunct to interpretation, it could never be a substitute for it."

With adolescent patients in particular, the reassurance intervention will have to be guarded against having the opposite effect from the one desired, which is, helping the patient to bear anxiety. For an illustration of an unwanted effect we might choose reassurance that sets off the conflict over time continuity. If we, for example, suggest that in time he may be less distressed about the failure of his examination or the loss of his girl friend, the patient may experience this not as reassurance but as a meaningless "putting off" statement, or as one young adult said in quoting a folk song: "work and pray, live on hay . . . you'll get pie in the sky when you die." This was the patient's way of asserting that to him the moment mattered, while the concept "in time" was vague and amorphous, without reality and certainly not any comfort to him.

This kind of reassurance for this patient would increase, rather than decrease, anxiety, which would have been the purpose of the intervention, in order to prepare the ground for a lasting interpretation. We should think of the patient's ability to make use of the kind of reassurance that is ego-syntonic for him, rather than offer a generalized statement to which he may be allergic.

As with later interpretations, with reassurances too we might be on safer ground if we—at least in the beginning—do not venture into sensitive areas but offer simple and direct acceptance of a painful state, without attempting to redirect or ameliorate the feeling which the patient has shared with us. Unless we can have compassion for the way in which the patient has experienced frustration, we cannot console or reassure him, and would do better to remain silent, for nothing interferes with positive transference more than an insincere or casual attempt at reassurance.

To the extent to which such suggestions as reassurance and similar interventions are steps leading to interpretations, we should take care to plan each step as sensitively as possible, since this will have a definite effect on the impact of an interpretation. Conversely, we might say that ineffective reassurances tend to increase resistances, particularly with patients who suffer from mild paranoid thinking disorders, and specifically with young adults who are always ready to withdraw to earlier role-playing acting-out attempts.

The awareness of all the adolescent characteristics may alert us to the many ways in which young adult patients may use our interpretations. Since it is axiomatic that patients will at times "misunderstand" something we have said and report aspects of a session in slightly distorted forms to friends, we can anticipate such defensive expressions with many of our young adult patients. We cannot completely avoid such distortions, but it is helpful if we hear what we say with the ear of the adolescent. The question "How will this interpretation sound to the patient, how will it come across to him—with his particular characteristics, over and above the individual character structure?" may make what we have to say more effective.

In the whole matter of language used for interpretation with our adolescent patients, several exceptions to the common practices seem indicated. While it is generally assumed that we talk in plain, nontechnical language to our patients, there is a question whether we may increase or decrease resistance with the young adult if we "snub" him by not using the technical terms that he is using. Partially as an expression of role-playing ("the good patient," the "intelligent young man"), partially as a result of their self-image crisis, many young adults tend to refer to their "super-ego," their "oedipus complex" or their "castration anxiety." If we asked them to define such terms fully, they will engage in an obsessional, hair-splitting definition bout, or they will fall silent, feeling that we are, as one patient put it, "pulling professional rank" or "putting me down." To substitute nontechnical descriptions ("your inner censor" for "super-ego") is likewise felt as editorial or educational criticism. We do not want to introduce lingo in our sessions, but it may speed up matters if we, at least in the opening phase, accepted the patient's need to sound informed and go along with his use of technical language without commenting.

Where we can make our insight felt is not so much in this aspect but in an insistence on not interpreting isolated words or actions, slips of the tongue, or any aspect of parapraxia. Whether the material comes from a dream or the report of realistic episodes, the young adult is often impressed with his "freudian slips," his "interesting forgetting" of names or terms or similar isolated phenomena. Not taking up these fragments is both realistically reassuring ("I don't have to watch every word I'm saying here") and clinically sound, since we do not want to be side-tracked into archaic aspects but wait until we have a solid theme on which we can comment with meaning. When the young adult needs to impress us with his intelligence, we can use this need to divert him from the tendency to be merely clever. For example, when he reports a very confusing and disorganized dream, we can react by asking whether he can see any theme in this bewildering material. The primary value of such an intervention is to help the patient to become used to our method of tracing themes as a basis for any sound interpretation.

When it comes to the question of timing of interpretations we may want to keep in mind the adolescent characteristic of time continuity, which may make it necessary to begin interpretations earlier in the session and in the analysis than we might be used to doing with adult patients who can cope with the frustration of waiting, as a factor of time continuity, better than some of our adolescents. This should not be interpreted as meaning overtalkativeness on the part of the analyst, but should be understood as another variation for this patient and this kind of analytic therapy. Short, compact interpretations that clearly hit the target and are based on sufficient data will usually be safer with the young adult than long and involved statements made toward the end of the session or after several months of association.

Because the adolescent tends to rely on his super-ego or his ego-ideals in coping with his resistances, he will often turn the analytic session into a learning situation and consider new intellectual knowledge as a sign of progress in treatment.

To cope with this defense, it seems particularly necessary to allow the adolescent patient ample time for "working through." When Freud first used this concept he said: "One must allow the patient time to become more conversant with the resistance . . . to *work through* it, to overcome it, by continuing, in defiance of it, the analytic work according to the fundamental rule of analysis . . ." (Novey, 1962). Since 1914, when this was written, a number of authors have stressed the parallel between mourning and working through, i.e., to correct faulty reality testing. There have been discussions about the necessity to treat "working through" as a special aspect of the therapeutic process.

In any case, the whole question of "working through" revolves around the effectiveness of insight, which has been described as a circular process, involving the ego and the self-image. Applied to the self-image crisis of the adolescent, we would expect recourse to the learning aspect of this process. The connection between affective experiences and learning theory, as emphasized by Novey (1962), suggests the temptation to fall back on passive wishes, which in turn will aid the resistance. For this reason alone, with the young adult it would seem important to withhold interventions or interpretations until he has reached the point where it becomes necessary for him to take the initiative and associate. This is one instance in which we cannot do anything but wait passively instead of trying to interpret the silence or any other aspect of the resistance. As Stewart suggested, the purpose of working through is not to accept the loss of a love object, as in mourning (passive), but to change the aims of the instinctual drives (active).

In reviewing the literature, Greenson arrived at a working definition of working through, by suggesting that "we do not regard the analytic work as working through before the patient has insight, only after. It is the goal of working through to make insight effective, i.e., to make significant and lasting changes in the patient. . . . "(1965).

Another area in which the young adult's tendency to use intellectual defenses may interfere with therapy is in his understanding of free association. As a rule, when we suggest to the young adult patient that he say whatever comes to his mind at the moment, he takes this as a request to verbalize his conscious thoughts. In fact, he explains his silences by saying, "I'm not thinking of anything." In other words, the emphasis is on thought, rather than on affect. We sometimes can help the patient with his stalemate by asking about his feelings at the moment as he experiences them consciously. This inquiry by itself may startle the patient who is under the impression that he should tell us something "new," events in his life between the last session and this one, something he did or said— all expressed in the familiar statement: "Nothing happened." Inquiry into feelings or fantasies, daydreams or partial affects may remove some of the super-ego barriers which are used in behalf of the resistances.

SPECIAL TECHNICAL PROBLEMS

The interplay of psychodynamic and socioeconomic factors which characterize post-adolescence frequently makes for some distinct difficulties in treatment that we usually do not encounter in working with younger adolescents or with adults.

We are referring to a number of interferences that are not psychologic in origin, but often become serious challenges to both the patient and the clinician. We tend in our work to view most of the material presented by the patient as psychologic in nature, just as we tend to think of the patient-clinician relationship as a transference manifestation. However, not all of the patient's expressions need to be based on transference, just as some of the problems presented may be an expression of objective reality disturbances, rather than a result of intra-psychic forces.

For an illustration of a realistic interference in therapy of the post-adolescent in particular, we may consider the issue of military training, to which young men in their late teens and early twenties are subject, and which, while predictable, nevertheless causes a severe disturbance, particularly when the country is involved in a war. Not only is the young adult at this age experiencing a profound disturbance in his personal life, his professional or vocational training, his relationship to those he loves, a reawakening of his identity crisis, and a heightening of all the adolescent characteristics, but society now expects him to experience new emotions: patriotism, love of country, hate of an enemy he has never seen, identification with men he has never seen, a readiness to sacrifice his own life—a life which he has barely begun to fathom. The therapy which he has finally started, after a long period of doubt and hesitation, is suddenly interrupted when his local draft board calls him, and the young adult now expects his therapist to protect him from experiences for which he usually is not in the least ready.

This natural expectation produces a set of related problems specific to the situation: it changes the patient-therapist relationship and transforms the analyst into an ally, a benign friend who writes letters to official sources, describing details from the analytic experience which he ordinarily would not share with anybody. This is bound to affect the transference, and create in the patient feelings of gratitude and, later, guilt over his hostile feelings.

The extramural contact with official sources—draft board, government sources—may at best postpone the interruption of treatment and give the young adult a deferred status. Many young people are concerned that this classification may interfere with future government or private employment. In many situations, letters from clinicians have been disregarded by selective service workers with the result that the patient's worst fears have been justified: his existing anxieties are heightened to a danger-ous level; in certain patients, homosexual panic does set in; suicidal and homicidal tendencies have become sharpened; reality testing has been weakened. That this is of no value to society is understood; what concerns us specifically is the effect of being drafted on young adults who should continue to be in therapy until they are well enough to function.

That certain patients who are not equipped to make the necessary reality adaptations have sought such escapes as flight into foreign countries, attempting to live anonymously, or have given up all attempts to adjust to reality is understandable. Between the time the first threat occurs in the life of the young adult until the final decision of his draft board, many months, perhaps a year, may pass. I have seen a number of patients regress sharply during this period with a reappearance of many symptoms. There have been more depressions, a return to hallucogenic experiences, a giving up of the struggle for success in work or study, a general loosening of controls. Therapy during such a waiting period is seriously hampered because the reality threat is constantly hanging over any attempt to explore or reconstruct aspects of earlier ego fractures.

In addition to these realistic environmental changes which affect the patient-therapist relationship during such a crisis, there is the constant danger of counter-transference manifestations interfering with our work. Over-identification and counter-hostility are both understandable reactions on our part, however slight or however well disguised. At the same time, the patient looks to us for constancy in behavior, as one of the few sane reality tests he has at this point of his life. That this situation demands more activity on our part—including the correspondence in our patients' behalf—than may be clinically indicated is still another aspect of special problems in our work with young adults.

Not all of these special problems present as drastic a situation as the one described, although they too require the therapist to employ a highly flexible and, at times, unconventional technique. Most of the challenges arise from the particular position of adolescents, in particular the overlapping of socioeconomic and psychodynamic factors.

Because the young adult is no longer an adolescent, is no longer living with his family and yet not completely self-sufficient economically, all questions relating to his income, financial management, and use of community resources tend to come up in the analytic hour. During the treatment process the therapist will be called upon to function at times as a social worker, then as a vocational guidance counselor, and then as a resource consultant.

Before we consider some of these specific situations, it might be well to recall once again that, by taking over these roles even temporarily, we are using essentially nonanalytical devices and resorting to the educational technique of exploiting the transference for reasons of expediency. That this will have an effect on the subsequent course of treatment, both transference and counter-transference manifestations, is understood. As soon as we adopt policies of guidance, we are interfering with the transference, and, for this reason alone, may want to weigh the current advantages of making a recommendation or offering a community resource against the disadvantages of later interferences in our analytic goals.

> For an illustration we may consider a gifted, attrac-
> tive young woman who tended to act-out impulsively,
> suggesting that she was postponing the end of role-playing
> throughout her adolescence and into post-adolescence. This
> was observable in study, employment, and heterosexual re-
> lationships. When the "escape into marriage" threatened
> both the continuation of therapy—her potential husband's
> permanent residence was in Europe—and the gains made in
> therapy, the analyst acted-out some of his counter-trans-
> ference by implying that this marriage could not work for
> the patient and would, in fact, interfere with all her realistic
> goals. While he was careful not to make direct suggestions,

his disapproval came across clearly to the patient, who correctly accused her therapist of acting like her father, even though she realized that he was more objective and thought only of her "own good."

There probably is no better evidence for the limitation of transference-authority results than that presented by this young woman who had fully cooperated with her therapist—and then got married during his vacation!

On the other side, there is the young adult from a rigid family who was so unable to handle his own finances— being careless as a sign of independence—that he was twice evicted from his living quarters and remained behind in his payments to his therapist for many months, without having made any arrangements for deferred payments. While the therapist had attempted to interfere with his patient's masochistic acting-out through appropriate interpretations, it became apparent after a time that much more reconstruction and remembering would be necessary before the patient could cope with reality. In the meantime, the patient was about to be asked to leave school because of nonpayment of tuition and had been threatened with a lawsuit by a department store. At this point, the analyst stepped out of his analytic role and functioned as a good social worker by helping his client to make a realistic budget—a totally new concept to the borderline patient. While the therapist was careful not to do more than was necessary in order for the young adult to experience the new idea of realistic planning of income and outgo over a period of time, he was nevertheless directing or guding his patient. Since he kept such activities to a very minimum without elaborating on them, the temporary detour into counseling proved helpful. It was significant that the therapist did not continue to help the patient resolve his budget problems in following sessions, but made it clear that the initial counseling had been, so to speak, an extracurricular activity which the young adult was perfectly capable of carrying on by himself. In other words, when the patient used this guidance activity in behalf of his resistances, bringing in more budget sheets, instead of free associating, the therapist checked himself and went on with the work of exploring, which he and his patient had undertaken to do together in the analytic process.

Altogether, the problem of the handling of money in the therapy of older adolescent patients tends to require a special technique. With adolescent patients, whose bills are paid by a family member, the subject of money seldom comes up in the psychoanalytic material, while, with adult patients, feelings about paying can be analyzed as part of the resistance. With young adults, often part of the bill is paid by the patient and the remainder by a family member. The situation may be complicated when the parents have been divorced and both parents contribute toward the therapy, each having attitudes differing from the other toward the son or daughter and the therapist. There are also many situations in which young people experiment with employment, changing jobs and going through periods of unemployment. Most therapists who work with young adults are well acquainted with the sudden cutting off of funds by a family member, threatening the interruption of therapy.

When a young graduate student on a tuition scholarship discovered, during the process of analytic exploration, that he was not doing his best work because he clearly was in the wrong field, he took steps to change his professional plans—steps which caused serious financial repercussions from his family, who still partially supported him and his therapy. It was indeed the patient's super-ego, based on an identification with his strong father, that had made him choose a career for which he was not suited. In retaliation, the father, as part of his competition both with son and therapist, cut off funds, creating a typical special problem in the treatment of young adults: both the intersection of the self-image dilemma with the economic bind, and the counter-transference. As with any interference by the community, government, or family, the analytic situation is disrupted, demanding more active measures than may be called for by clinical necessity.

The punitive abandonment by the father may increase all of the basic conflicts of the patient; in particular, it will heighten, rather than resolve, the self-image dilemma, the identity diffusion, and the hesitation to give up role-playing. For a period, withdrawal and mild depression may be expected, while the transference hangs in the balance. If the patient is to continue treatment, he will need the good will and trust of his therapist, a situation which has to have an effect on the self-image dilemma and his ability to associate freely in the future, particularly when he experiences both homosexual and hostile feelings.

The therapist, professionally obliged to continue with an ongoing case, is *nolens volens* put in the position of the "better father," a role he does not want to have in an analytic relationship.

There is the unrealistic possibility of interrupting or ending treatment, which will be experienced by the patient as abandonment by both father and therapist. It will undo many of the therapeutic gains, since such a solution will mean to the patient that the therapist was interested in him only as long as father paid for the therapy, making father right, and may then tip the self-image dilemma in favor of the punitive, hostile super-ego—which had brought him into therapy in the first place, when he discovered that he had chosen the wrong professional career to please father.

In practice, the responsible clinician has hardly any other choice than to go on with the case and analyze his own resistances by himself, since this kind of situation will produce both aggressive counter-transference and counter-resistance feelings in the therapist.

A different kind of characteristic young adult problem arises for the therapist and his analytic relationship to his patient when the adolescent, who has begun to set up his own home and style of life, inquires about community resources and wants reliable advice from his therapist for referral to a physician, a dentist, or a gynecologist.

As in the analysis of adults, we want to examine all requests for advice as possible transference resistances, which aim to prevent production of memories by re-enacting childhood situations in the transference. At the same time, we want to remember that requests for advice may also be based on ignorance or lack of experience in the adult world. There would be, for example, a considerable difference between a young woman patient who claims not to use birth control methods because "I don't know where to go," and the patient who is ready to practice birth control but has not had the opportunity to find a reliable gynecologist in the town to which she has only recently moved. Since the girl who had recently moved into the town did not want to discuss her problem with her colleagues at school, with whom she was not on intimate terms, and did not know any people whose opinion she felt she could trust, the request for information from her analyst seemed to have a realistic basis.

There may be justification for giving certain factual information, particularly about community resources, to young adults. Both the insistence on analyzing every request of the patient and the eagerness to "steer" him to the best source may be an expression of anxiety on the therapist's part.

There are a great many small and large details of daily life with which the young adult is not familiar, having been overprotected, or having avoided his family as a natural source of information. Once our young adult patient is 21 years old, he or she is legally responsible for signing a lease, buying on installment, and making verbal, binding working agreements. Because some young adults are no-toriously inexperienced, they will at times be exploited by irresponsible businessmen—situations which, when multi-plied, are bound to be harmful to their growing sense of independence and self-confidence. Again, as with other nonanalytic communications, we will have to guard against acting-out the counter-transference and become the "better, protecting parent" when we subtly suggest that the young adult call the housing department if the landlord refuses to return his rent deposit. The question of whether or not to give this kind of casual advice or guid-ance will be encountered often when treating young adults, and while we would not like to see our young adult patients hurt, due to lack of experience, we will have to consider the price we pay for this kind of friendly guidance in terms of the more basic goals of analytic therapy. From the experience of a number of clinicians who have worked with adolescents it would appear that suggestions made in the opening phase of therapy will more seriously interfere with analytic work than those made during the middle or end phase, when there is emphasis on working through rather than uncovering and remembering.

The above applies as well to the occasional acting-out in adolescence, particularly when it involves identification with reference groups who interfere with the analytic work. As with other interferences, we will be tempted to use guidance or authority to stem the tide of regressive, primary thinking and pleasure-principle behavior. This will occur after our more usual interventions have failed, owing to either the stickiness of the patient's libido or untimely faulty interpretations. Just as we do not like to see a young adult make foolish, long-range commitments, we will regret his joining groups in which he takes LSD, gets involved in drug-pushing, or other illegal activities, or, as one group proposed, take the law into their own hands and steal what they desire from homes of wealthy acquaintances or relatives. Some clinicians, after having failed with both interpretations and suggestions, have used authority by telling the young adult that unless he stops this acting-out behavior, they cannot continue working with him. One therapist threatened to commit his patient to a psychotic ward after having told him that he was not capable of using good judgment by himself.

This is, of course, a long way from analytic therapy and possibly represents an acting-out of unrecognized negative counter-transference, which is just as damaging to treatment as any acting-out by the patient.

There may, on rare occasions, be room for the use of transference authority. However, as with suggestions or referrals to resources, this could not be effective until quite late in the treatment process, when we can be certain that disapproval will have an—even temporary—impact on the patient and will be worth the price in increased resistance in the transference. Above all, we would have to be sure that the patient needs this kind of educational intervention.

> To illustrate this type of use of authority, we will consider a young adult who, after several hundred hours of therapy, went into a slump and regressed markedly, using poor reality testing and increasing anxiety to a dangerous point. The material in the sessions at that time consisted of the patient reporting his complex problems in graduate school, as well as in his place of employment. When he mentioned that he had found a solution to his troubles by intending to sign a lease for a store with some unusual merchandise, instead of keeping his present job and continuing to study, the therapist detected a clear note of doubt in the patient's voice and felt that the young adult, as he later admitted, "wanted to be talked out of this nonsense." The therapist used his authority at this crucial time to ask the patient not to sign any long-term lease until he was quite clear what this would mean for his future in the long

run. While the request was made in the form of a strong suggestion, the clinician had been using transference authority, being convinced that this was a moment when he had no other choice. The indication for the use of this form of guidance came from the fact that the patient brought the material not in a regular session but by a phone call, explaining that if he signed the lease, this would have to be done before the next session.

Since the therapist well knew the forms that depersonalization episodes and identity diffusions took in this patient, he could afford to intervene promptly without marked damage to the later treatment relationship. That the young adult took the unusual step of calling by phone was his way of asking to be stopped from acting-out.

In clinical terms, one might well raise the question whether or not the therapist's suggestion aided or hindered the resolution of the self-image dilemma: the patient was at this point struggling with the development of a more realistic ego-ideal, against the pseudoideal which had originally beem promoted by his schizoid mother who exploited his narcissism and greatly increased his omnipotent fantasies.

To sign the store lease and "become rich quick" would have been acting out the pseudoideal. From all indications it seemed very unlikely that this patient could have financially survived or succeeded in this venture. Whether the economic failure would have strengthened his reality sense is a matter of speculation, since, in fact, he did not go through with his scheme. From all indications of the patient's past history, it is quite possible that he would have learned nothing from a possible failure and financial loss, but would have blamed outside forces for his misfortune. At least this is how he rationalized his previous failures. The ability to learn from mistakes depends on the capacity of the ego to critically examine one's actions without overreaction or rationalization. For this reason it seems likely that the therapist's protective gudance at this one moment bypassed the potential of economic upset and perhaps allowed the patient and his therapist to stay close to the significant core of the problem: the ego of the patient, which is, after all, the final test of all our efforts.

REFERENCES:

Arlow, J. A., and Brenner, Ch. (1964): *Psychoanalytic Concepts and the Structural Theory*. International Universities Press, New York, pp. 28 and 81.

Berliner, B. (1958): The role of object relations in moral masochism. Psychoanal. Quart. 27: 38–56.

Freud, S. (1958): Remembering, Repeating and Working Through. Standard Edition 12. Hogarth Press, California. pp. 145–156.

Glover, E. (1955A): *Technique of Psychoanalysis*. International Universities Press, New York.

Glover, E. (1955B): *Technique of Psychoanalysis*. A Questionnaire Research. International Universities Press, New York, p. 276.

Greenacre, Ph. (1952): The predisposition to anxiety. In: *Trauma, Growth and Personality*. N. N. Norton, New York.

Greenson, R. (1965): The problem of working through. In: *Drives, Affects and Behavior*, Vol. 2, M. Schur, Ed. International Universities Press, New York, pp. 277–313.

Lewin, B., and Ross, H. (1960): *Psychoanalytic Education in the U. S.* Norton & Co., New York.

Menninger, K. (1958): *Theory of Psychoanalytic Technique*. Basic Books, New York, p. 30.

Novey, S. (1962): The principle of working through in psychoanalysis. J. Amer. Psychoanal. Assoc. 10:658–676.

Nunberg, H. (1955): *Principles of Psychoanalysis*. International Universities Press, New York, p. 122.

Schmideberg, M. (1935): Reassurance as a means of analytic technique. Int. J. Psychoanal. 16: 474–499.

Schur, M. (1953): The ego and anxiety. In: *Drives, Affects and Behavior*. International Universities Press, New York.

Stewart, W. (1963): An inquiry into the concept of working through. J. Amer. Psychoanal. Assoc. 11: 474–499.

Zetzel, E. (1949 and 1953): Anxiety and the capacity to bear it, and depression and the incapacity to bear it. In: *Drives, Affects and Behavior*. International Universities Press, New York.

Section III

YOUTH AND SOCIETY

Chapter 11

YOUTH AND COMMUNITY: AN INTERVIEW WITH MAXWELL JONES

It is remarkable that in spite of the one-sided view that is so forcefully presented through the long years of medical training that one could escape from accepting the medical authoritarian hierarchical model as the only way of looking at doctor-patient relationships. It is precisely this that Dr. Jones has been able to achieve. He established a unit for treating psychopaths in England in 1946, where patients participated in all decisions affecting the unit, a treatment approach which is now known as therapeutic community.

He believes that most institutions in our society are built on authoritarian hierarchical systems. Hospitals are organized and run by staff who neither attempt to obtain nor pay any attention to any feedback from those it purports to serve. This, he believes, is also true of our schools, colleges and universities.

It is with this perspective that he looks at the problems of youth, the violence at campuses, school dropouts, and developing of communes, all resulting from a lack of two-way communication and sharing of decision making. He believes that youth today are struggling and fighting to get what society, if it were wise, should be offering them without their asking—a real opportunity to participate.

Question: Let me ask you as a psychiatrist who is

interested in social sciences, how do you understand the problems of youth today?

Maxwell Jones: Well, it's a global question, and I will speak very subjectively. When I was trying to get close to the young adults in London, working at the Henderson Hospital, we had to say, "We do not know how to help you; you've got to help us to find out how to help, and how to get close to you. You dislike authority, you dislike seniority, then let us try to structure a society, the contemporary kind where we live 24 hours a day; where we share the responsibility, where we listen to each other, and let us see what emerges." We found that we needed interpreters. We realized that unless these people were prepared to be their own interpreters so that they could bring the ecological dimension into our understanding of what it was like to live in the east end of London, we were not going to understand the problems. Our goal was to help people to help themselves and not to do something for them in the professional sense.

Question: People are saying that the youth today are alienated; would you like to comment on it?

Maxwell Jones: I think that our models in society are all built on the authoritarian hierarchical system. Although we talk about society in democracy we don't understand it in practice. When we look at hospitals we see no real attempt, in Europe or America, to trust patients, who can really do a lot for themselves. This can also be seen in the school system and the university system everywhere. We draw the assumption that the older you are, the more senior you are, the more you know and the more right you have to determine attitudes and values for other people, and I think that this alienates the youngster with any wish to have individuality. He doesn't want to fit into these molds; that is obvious, but the obvious isn't always obvious.

Question: Our generation was not brought up as democratically as the present youth generation. Why didn't we feel alienated, and why is this present generation so alienated from society?

Maxwell Jones: Well, we're getting into all kinds of imponderables. First of all, the tempo of society is quickening at an alarming rate. A person can barely keep up with it. The industrial revolution was easy because it gave you time to accommodate to the changes that were occurring. It is different when we get into the so-called computer age or whatever you call it. In the past we could learn history and we could apply it in a way that meant something. Now I don't think history could mean a sausage to a young person because past history has little to do with life during the present era and there are no guidelines. We have almost got to start all over again and I am sure that this is what the violence and the revolutionary elements are all about. Young people are looking for a totally new value system. I have a lot of sympathy for them.

Let me explain by something I am involved in at present. I've just come from a school where we are trying to establish a therapeutic community (Jones 1953) with 13-year-olds, which is an easy place to start. In the class there will be six adults and twenty children. I am finding that to get them to look at behavior and examine it in an open-minded way is infinitely easier than to try to develop a similar system in an organization such as Fort Logan Mental Health Center. It is difficult because professional people have concepts, attitudes and ideas of power and status. These are not there in a 13-year-old class. We are able to discuss subjects like the effect of people on other people and the subject of authority and leadership.

People have often wondered why, in our society, leaders do not emerge who have the confidence to confront the authority system with what it is doing. Politicians and businessmen get away with murder because their bluff works and no one thinks that you can confront the system except some students and hippies. The students today are learning that teachers are not always right and the Establishment can be success-fully challenged. They are beginning to look at the new philosophy of education in which there is a striking difference between teaching and learning. Everybody in my age group at least got teaching but no learning. I learned nothing at university; I wasn't expected to be involved or to have an opinion; I was just supposed to be a sponge. Now this is changing. I think we are in a stage of evolution, sometimes revolution, where the whole idea of change is becoming a way of life.

Question: Are you saying that the confrontations on the university campuses are a good thing?

Maxwell Jones: I'm saying that this is a leaderless, as yet unstructured, mass of people. They know vaguely that they want a more important place in the administrative and decisional structure and I have every sympathy with their wanting to be involved in a situation. I have great belief in structure, if the structure is properly balanced so that everyone listens to everyone else and an appropriate amount of time is devoted to interaction, with experienced leadership providing direction. If this direction leads to action and action leads to change and learning then it is part of the ongoing process of education.

We have the principal of a university who has forgotten what it is like to be a student. We as doctors ideally should live in the community we serve, but if we can't do that then we have to have mediators or interpreters from that culture. Our involvement, if it can't be personal, must be through some mediator who is personally involved, such as a "nonprofessional." Then we can get something of a blend of the skills of the professional, who has been trained in a particular area, together with the earthy awareness of the person who is in the system or who is in the situation. It is in that way that I see learning theories coming into their own. But we have to have adequate structure if all this is to take place.

Question: You mean structure within the university?

Maxwell   Structure within whatever system, and this
Jones: is the area that has been totally inadequate up to now. In an organization we have skilled people, but their social organization is lousy. There is an attempt at democracy, but it is essentially bureaucracy; there is little trust for the delegation of responsibilities and authority, and this does not produce leaders. A leader only emerges in action. You just cannot create leaders sitting around and talking. They have got to demonstrate their leadership quality in action.

If you were to say to me, "Look there's a hell of a stink on the campus of a university," whom could you recommend to go in as the facilitator? Whom would you think of? It wouldn't be anyone in the university structure; it wouldn't be anyone in the student body; in all probability, it would have to be someone who has a very wide perspective in group dynamics, in authority structure, and in the ecology.

Question: So you are depending a great deal on the quality of leadership?

Maxwell Jones: Definitely. That goes without saying; and the quality implies much more than neutrality. It implies a capacity to blend the various elements so that a process of learning is initiated. This is where I would be hard put to think of any name that I am aware of who has this capacity to be an active leader and at the same time to be impersonal. Working, not with any self-gain, not with any hidden motives, but by really looking at himself as a facilitator of the learning process. This is an area where, as yet, we are green.

Question: Let me ask you a more direct question: How would you deal with a campus crisis, if you were the president of a university?

Maxwell Jones: Well, I can give you a concrete example that is just in the planning stage. The University of Colorado in Colorado Springs wants to establish a student health service, and they asked me for help. I, with a colleague of mine, went there and we listened to the three people who would be concerned in the psychologic field. They had no clear ideas of how to involve the students and so we went a stage further and said, "Well, if we were going to be involved, we would want the students to decide on the kind of health service they wanted." From the start, the planning would be built around the consumer and his needs. We think that the person establishing such a service would probably be better without an office, that he would be simply part of the university life and available for informal communications. He would then say, "Well, who are your buddies, and would you like to bring them along?" This would extend to their whole social set, their social system and their family system. And it would be a system built up from the individual and his peers. There is nothing new about this. It is ordinary theory, or whatever you would like to call it, but it means that the facilitator would help the student and his peer group, his family and his outside complex to become involved in the problem with a view to changing the system so that it would alter his own image of himself. On the other hand, if I take your example, which is a bit more difficult, I would follow the same set of principles that we worked out in Scotland where we asked for a facilitator so that opposing forces could come together immediately with no waiting and no waste of time because the learning is greatest when the interest is greatest. At this point I would say, "Well, who would you like as a facilitator, or what persons would you like to help this process, assuming that they were aware of the possible advantages of such a procedure?" Within a hospital you can get that awareness, but in a university this situation is newer. I think that it would have a sort of universal validity that you want to have noninvolved, objective, trained people without identification for either side to facilitate the process. Now if the opposing forces can decide on a suitable person whom they could trust, who would not be biased, who would have a public image of a very formidable kind, then you've made the first step in the right direction, because you've initiated the trust and you established the structure which will allow the process to continue.

Question: That sounds interesting because, as far as I can remember, during the various campus crises very serious efforts were made between the administration and the students to get together, but I don't think that they brought in somebody from outside.

Maxwell Jones: Well that is an important step, but the biggest problem would be to find people with that kind of strength and skill and interest, because it could be dangerous. I would hesitate personally if I were asked to act in the role of a facilitator, let us say between youth groups at one of the local high schools where there has been violence. I would be a bit scared because the question of actually getting the two groups to listen, when the tension is so high, may be impossible. One might have to use some cooling off period before one could actually utilize this process.

Question: In your book *Beyond the Therapeutic Community* (Jones, 1968) you have emphasized certain principles, such as two-way communication, decision by consensus, the importance of social learning. Now there are reports that some young people have dropped out of society and have established communes in the countryside, where they are living together and sharing everything. Do you think that these people in an unsophisticated way are trying to establish a therapeutic community?

Maxwell Jones: I think so. I think that there are all kinds of models. The Kibbutz, of course, comes to mind and I think that in a much wider perspective there are religious orders. All these are attempts at having people come together with certain expectations and means to develop a system. If you take a commune where there is sharing of property and skills, then it might well be that values can be modified considerably. Within such a value system my awareness is that artistic products, which are made commercial ventures, can be seen as not necessarily a financial reward system but as satisfaction for one's actual image of oneself for one's own creative ability. I gather that some communes managed to do this, and I think that this is fascinating. This is one of the positive things that I have learned from my research of the past 12 years, that not everybody is bitten by this money incentive or with this idea of power. This is something that is indoctrinated in the schools, and this is one of the things that I am trying to get at, by working with young people in the school.

My experience has been that values can be changed in a remarkably short time, in a group that has certain things in common. There must be some common interest and some common goal to make such a group cohesive, otherwise there is no homogeneity. I think one can talk about various pockets of society with their own particular value system. That's what a therapeutic community is—it's an unreal microcosm of society; it's a transitional community for the purpose of learning, learning how to live, learning how to relate, learning how to improve your image of yourself, and these are not material goals. There are many examples of this. The drug addiction field is one, where the therapeutic potential of the peer group has been clearly shown. These are really therapeutic communities.

Question: You were talking about a hospital, as compared to a university. You have been the superintendent at Dingleton Hospital in Scotland, how far do you think you succeeded in establishing a therapeutic community there?

Maxwell Jones: Well, I am at present involved in writing my assessment of the changes that took place over a 7-year period during which I was superintendent of Dingleton Hospital. My own goals were clear enough. I took on this powerful role in order to be able to sanction change because to have power at the top is the best way to bring about change. These 7 years have confirmed all my beliefs, that, by slowly helping people to believe that their combined efforts are far better than those of any one authority figure, one can move from a typical authority structure to a multiple leadership structure in a multi-disciplinary setting. In that system it would have been impossible for me to make a unilateral decision because it would have been totally outside the expectations of the culture built up, where shared decision-making was an absolute necessity. Once a structure is set up, then this process has its own dynamics and needs very little direction. I think I was the last medical superintendent at Dingleton. Even in a rigid structure of a mental hospital under the National Health Service we now have a structure of six formal leaders: three from the medical profession, the head of social work, the head of nursing and the hospital administrator. Six people share the formal responsibility; this degree of change within 7 years isn't bad.

Question: What about the patients, do they share any authority?

Maxwell Jones: I don't think that we have developed that much. The staff began to learn and began to get interested in their own development and growth. I found that this was something of a problem. Before I left Dingleton

we were beginning to have a bad conscience about the extent to which we were
getting movement with the staff and
relatively less movement in the patients,
partly because we were putting our own
interest first. There is also the question of
how far a patient body can go. I don't know.
I do know that at Henderson we took them
much further than we ever did at Dingleton.
The patients at Henderson were sociopaths,
and, as you know, among sociopaths there
often are some very creative thinkers;
these you don't encounter in a hospital with
geriatric and psychotic patients.

Question: Do you think that one could introduce
similar changes in a university administrative structure?

Maxwell
Jones: Yes, I think that it should be much easier
theoretically, because, in the university,
people are supposed to be interested in
change; whether or not they are, in fact, is
another matter.

Question: I would assume from what you said that
you would be supportive of student representation in the administrative structure
of the university. Do you see any dangers of
this process going too far?

Maxwell
Jones: Sure, and the dangers are largely in the
area of learning. Somehow we have got to
bridge this gap from the revolutionary,
wildly hitting out, to the developmental
process, which will mean generations of

student control and a culture which becomes ingrained in the whole system. But I think this would take a decade of trial and error and growing of skill and responsibility amongst the student body. It is a long process.

Question: Some people are saying that we have all these problems with the young not necessarily because it is a computer age and not because technical changes have taken place, but because we brought up these kids permissively; would you like to comment on that?

Maxwell Jones: I do not think that the trouble we are having with our young is necessarily having bad results. I think the Sorbonne is a better place for the violence, which forced the power structure to realize that it could be overturned and which provided the motivation for a compromise. This is part of the process of change.

Question: But your generation and my generation didn't challenge the authority. We accepted a university as it was and we accepted the medical school as it was. Why is this generation rebelling and challenging and protesting?

Maxwell Jones: I haven't thought about it, but it is a good question. When I think of my youth, I myself rebelled against the system but only after I got every degree that I could get and had acceptance as a scholar or as a professional, which made it safe for me to rebel. Now people feel confident to rebel without that kind of support; I just don't know why that is.

Question: You don't think it could be attributed to affluence, that people don't fear starvation?

Maxwell Jones: Well, this is obvious and the movement is based upon a different value system, but how it came about I don't know.

Question: Do you feel that some principles of a therapeutic community approach could be applied to bringing up children in a family, such as two-way communication, shared decision-making?

Maxwell Jones: It would depend very much on the age of the children. I tried this kind of thing with my little girls, ages 6 to 12, and it just did not work. They were bored with discussion; they wanted to be told; they were not yet ready to assume the responsibility for their own decisions. So the usefulness of these principles depends very much on the age of the children.

Question: Let us look at business; a lot of young people are moving into business, and some of them are going into the business world to change it. Do you think that the principles of the therapeutic community can be applied in large corporations?

Maxwell Jones: I feel fairly confident about that. My experience has been that it is infinitely easier to talk to business people than to psychiatrists about subjects such as shared responsibility, joint decisions and two-way communication.

My contact with business has been through government committees. I was on a national committee, for instance, in London and I was appalled by the ineptitudes. There could be an obvious split between the chairman and the vice-chairman but none would dream of mentioning it; no one would have the skill to touch on it because it would take them away from the formal agenda and to look at the hidden agenda would be completely outside their confines.

In business you have two consumers: you have the person who buys the stuff, but then you have the staff at the lower levels. The opportunities for changing the buyer are infinitely less because he is not within a system, but the system under which the employee works does allow the change to reach him. One of the frustrating things is that change is in essence easy to bring about with the knowledge that we already have, but there are so few change agents around.

Question: Who is the change agent?

Maxwell Jones: The person with the authority and techniques: people who are brought in as consultants, people who could provide inspirational leadership.

Question: In your book you mention that our educational system does not provide social learning in any organized manner. Could you describe a way we could introduce social learning in our schools and universities?

Maxwell Jones: At present I am involved in a local school in an attempt to provide social learning and I think we are getting nearer to our goal. This is a class in a quite progressive school where we have a positive rapport with the principal. Besides myself, there are two councillors, a psychologist and two teachers involved in this experiment. All that we are doing is saying to the class that we have no agenda, that we simply want to talk about living, about life. The students were, of course, at first nonplussed because they had come to expect an e xplicit lesson and they are still wanting us to play the role of the teacher, but they are much closer to understanding that we are not going to be forced into this role of the teacher but that we want to be facilitators and to help them to help themselves.

We have had fairly predictable self-conscious discussions on prejudice and religion. The students talked of the heterosexual problem but they kept it away from sex. Last time, one of the teachers, who is in on this experiment, shared his failure to control his class and three of these 15-year-olds volunteered to go to the class with him. They went and the results were very satisfactory; their mere presence changed the situation. We spent the day discussing why these three youngsters, who are only one grade ahead of the class they went to, had this effect. We discussed the probability that they gave the class a feeling of importance in that another class of older students was interested in them, that their teacher was so concerned that he invited them to come. We then went on to look at this process and at the feedback. Half the class was bored because they hadn't been involved and showed some resentment towards the trio of "facilitators." We then asked, why were these people seen as somewhat alien? Obviously they had selected themselves; they got approval from the older persons; there was the beginning of rivalry. Later we discussed the reasons why the three facilitators, who are comparative outsiders, could have such impact on the class and lessen the quarreling and help the listening and interaction. Couldn't one do that in his own class. This is a tough question, because then that leads the more articulate people into saying, "Well I don't know if anyone would listen to us. We are too well-known." Then the class gave the example of their families—how they were not listened to in the family because there everyone knew everyone's point of view and it was just repetitious, and that the introduction of a stranger could make a difference. Here, we are getting at the whole idea of process and becoming aware of oneself; now this is getting closer to social learning as I see it.

Question: Are you suggesting that we should have facilitators going into the schools and bringing about these changes or are you suggesting that we should have different kinds of teachers who could act as facilitators as well.

Maxwell Jones: That would be the long-term ideal, but in the meantime we are kind of stuck with this need to train on the job, because the teachers aren't ready for this nor are we. I'm learning as much as the kids are learning. I find it a very rich experience and because I am learning and because the kids can see me as their peer in that sense, they are sharpening their teeth and they are attacking me quite a lot because they feel I have sanctioned it. This is a very good experience that adults can be pupils, that there can be a role reversal. Thinking is beginning to emerge leading to an analysis of leadership. Are the teachers really as great as they think they are? Must one conform? What happens if one does not conform? We are getting obvious instances of leaders emerging in this class. One boy is so good at developing blushes when he speaks, but he is becoming articulate and listening and the class is amazed that he is not only speaking but that they want to hear him and therefore we are getting both sides of the experience: what the group is doing with him and what he is doing in testing out his own capacity.

Question: Now when you said that you were being attacked, you were attacked by students. Now what about being attacked by the teachers, because here you are going in somebody else's territory; school is the territory of the teachers and you are obviously not a teacher in the orthodox sense. Now, are you being attacked by the teachers as a person who is coming in from ontside?

Maxwell Jones: Luckily the teacher in this class, a woman named Barbara, is very interested in this experiment, and so is the principal of this school. Barbara is forever trying to protect me. Today, when the kids were criticizing me, she tried to protect me by saying that they didn't pick up my point. At this, she was immediately jumped on by one of the adult peers who said that she was making value judgments and devaluing the children. This interaction showed the children that adults are able to attack each other and also provided a learning situation for Barbara.

Question: So you are suggesting that at this stage if one wants to promote social learning, then the first step would be to have facilitators going into the school and setting up models, the way you are doing in this particular experiment.

Maxwell
Jones:
That is right, and also incorporating the whole system to include the parents which, I think, is going to be fascinating because our feedback shows that the parents like what is happening very much.

Question:
Do you support the system of examinations that we have in the schools in testing and assessing knowledge?

Maxwell
Jones:
Oh God, no, I am more for growth than for learning, although obviously you have got to complement one with the other, but there is far too much emphasis on the side of teaching rather than on the side of learning. I am convinced that if schools are an apprenticeship in living, we should handle every "here and now" situation as a learning situation. Then I think that we could catch up with the computer age.

Question:
Taking social learning as one of the premises of the therapeutic community approach, you also say that "much treatment in psychiatry could just as well be called social learning" (Jones, 1953). Would you like to comment on this?

Maxwell
Jones:
When a person is put in a mental hospital and is diagnosed as sick, we are giving him the role of a sick person. The social role of a patient is to be ill and to be looked after. This reinforces dependency and helplessness, although some people need to be protected from the world for a time, but I feel that the basic problem is one of

adequacy in meeting the expectations of the social system.

Question: I get the feeling that you do not like the word "sick."

Maxwell Jones: No, I don't.

Question: If a person has emotional problems and he needs help and you won't call him sick, how would you go about labeling him and what would you do for him?

Maxwell Jones: I would prefer to call him a social casualty within a system, but one has to examine the system. We have very little skill in doing this but at least we do know one or two things. For instance, we know that when somebody has been identified as the patient by the system, then every effort is made to extrude him from the system, but, if at the time, instead of putting a finger on one person, one decides to see the whole family, it is with a clear understanding that one considers it a breakdown of the family. Very often, one person is singled out by the family as the cause of all the trouble and he is then brought to the psychiatrist so that a social crisis is changed into a medical emergency. The person's ability to fight back and stand up to the family is further impaired by his being labeled as mentally sick. After identifying someone as a patient and putting a diagnostic label on him, you further this process because then everything that he does is loaded in the direction of the medical staff's expectations. He has been called schizophrenic and therefore everything is directed towards this type of self-fulfilling prophecy. I think that we have really got to look at the system. It is a medical system, not a social system, or at least not a socially conscious system.

Question: How do you see the future role of the psychiatrist? You have stated that "by involving ourselves with social problems that are not directly related to mental disease we run the risk of being criticized on the grounds that we are exceeding the function of psychiatry." If we are not to exceed the function of psychiatry and if we are going to prove useful in this computer age, how do you see the psychiatrist's role in the future?

Maxwell Jones: Well I think that we probably ought to have another branch of psychiatry which is, in a sense, happening with social psychiatry, although a social psychiatrist should have a different type of training and a different function. It seems pretty obvious that either we will limit ourselves to sickness, which is a medical role, or we will have, as the young, action-oriented people want, another model, another system, in which total attention will not be centered on diagnosis, prognosis and medical criteria, but on playing a humble but significant part in the total social system.

Question: You say humble part, what do you mean?

Maxwell Jones: Well, it could mean a model where the psychiatrist is a resource person and comes in when somebody is considered as ill. But the training of such a psychiatrist would be different. He would have the skill to act as a facilitator between people.

Question: In a number of cities the young people are setting up youth clinics because some of the young people are refusing to go to hospitals, even to the out-patient departments, so they are going to community clinics, which are almost run by young people who get volunteer psychiatrists, physicians and medical students to staff them. How do you feel about this development?

Maxwell Jones: The lesson from developments of this nature is clear—that the medical model has failed. It does not have the flexibility to include social problems which constitute the bulk of present-day psychiatry. In spite of experiences with drug addicts and alcoholics, we still do not recognize the importance of help given by the peer group. I think the ultimate goal in psychiatry has to be to help people live within the system and within the law, but we are not going to stay in that system because we never were in it. All we can do is to be resource people and help the people within the system to help themselves. I know a clinic such as you describe that is run by a social worker. I have visited the clinic and I found the experience delightful. At the clinic they disregard all the rules; if they have very little money, they go to an auction and somehow still manage to get whatever equipment they want. It is their place; it is their plan. They have involved the society by having volunteer councillors. This is bringing in the peer group in a very positive way and in significant figures; this is community psychiatry. The people at the clinic are learning from professionals, whom they have as consultants, with whom they have frequent meetings, but, of course, the professionals are learning just as much about values and about life within that community. I think that somehow we have got to prevent those extreme professional and nonprofessional organizations, whose members want to exclude the other group. I think we need to experiment with an open mind, without the rigid convictions that powerful academic medical centers have, who pretend to accomplish a great deal but, in fact, accomplish little.

Question: The thing that interests me is that you are a physician by training and you went through medical school, which has a very structured hierarchical system. What made you think of the "therapeutic community" approach?

Maxwell Jones: Because I was totally sick of abuse of authority. I found that in medicine the system was considered more important than the patient as a person and the system was, of course, designed to meet the needs of the staff and not of the patient. I wanted to build something around the needs of the patient and here I was lucky that I had the opportunity.

Question: I still want to know, that having gone through the medical training, why were you not "brain-washed" like the rest of us into accepting the medical model?

Maxwell Jones: What really got me upset, and dissatisfied with the medical model was what I saw at Maudsley, where I worked as an assistant. The staff had a smug, self-centered contented attitude toward running the hospital for their own purposes. Teaching and research had a high priority compared to the patient and his welfare. This motivated me to rebel and I decided to try to develop a system which was patient-centered and not staff-centered.

Question: Would you say that you had been a rebel all your life and this was a sort of manifestation of your rebellion?

Maxwell Jones: Well I was a conformist rebel for 10 years until I felt strong enough to drop my conformity. I think that this must be part of my upbringing because my brother, who is a judge in Edinburgh, was the most rebellious member of the Scottish bar and has always been respected and sought out by groups because he would always take up causes. My mother had to strive hard to make ends meet. My parents were kind of religious, and went their own way rather than conform to materialistic standards. I think it was this home environment which influenced me to become very aware of the needs of others and question some of the accepted practices.

Question: You talked earlier about the importance of leadership. Would you expound on it, in relation to the present needs of our society?

Maxwell Jones: From my experiences I have learned that the more effective I felt as a leader, the more I found that the group was involved in the decision-making process. In my leadership roles, I have not knowingly taken any unilateral decision, because I am so totally convinced that no decision is worth anything unless it reflects the attitudes of the people who are going to implement it and who are going to be affected by it. If this principle is recognized and practiced by most people in leadership roles, such as university presidents, school principals, hospital superintendents and so on, then we would be on the threshold of a new and truly democratic society.

REFERENCES

Jones, M. (1953): *The Therapeutic Community.* Basic Books, New York.
Jones, M. (1968): *Beyond the Therapeutic Community: Social Learning and Social Psychiatry.* Yale University Press, New Haven.

Chapter 12

YOUTH IN CONFLICT: AN EXPLANATION BASED ON THE DEVELOPMENTAL APPROACH

S. Jalal Shamsie

The recent unrest in the universities, the increasing participation of the young in political activities and the challenging of the law by them, on an individual basis and collectively, have led society to wonder what ails our youth. Participation in the Civil Rights Movement was only the beginning of young people taking an active interest in the socio-political affairs. Since then, there has been strong opposition to the United States Government on the Vietnam issue, burning of draft cards, and open confrontation with the police, both in the streets and on the university campuses. This sudden student activism, which has not been confined solely to the North American continent but engulfs the whole of the Western World, has left society wondering about the nature and the causes of this unrest. Even the liberal elements of society, who are in sympathy with many of the demands and attitudes of the young, are apprehensive about the occasional irrational and violent mood that the youth protest has taken.

THE OLD CONFLICT

Before looking at any explanation of the question: "Why is youth in conflict with society?" let us define more clearly the nature of this conflict. The conflict we are concerned with is not the historical conflict which has existed since time immemorial between youth and the Establishment, where the vigor, energy and historical idealism of youth have always come into conflict with the need of the Establishment to maintain the status quo. It is a historical fact that the evolution of society has largely been due to social changes which were carried through by the young.

The older generation has always been disdainful of the young and has always held youth to be irresponsible and ungrateful. The following quotation illustrates this point:

> I see no hope for the future of our people if they are dependent on the frivolous youth of today, for certainly we were taught to be discreet and respectful of elders, but the present youth are exceedingly wise and impatient of restraint.
> —Hesiod, 8th century B.C.—

The conflict which has existed between the young and the older generation from early history has a useful function in the evolution of a society. The older generation, having arrived at certain goals, always desires stability and resists change. However, changes are necessary for the growth and evolution of a society and the young with their vigor, energy and idealism are best suited to help this come about. The young generally do not have the responsibilities that adults must be concerned with and have very little to lose since they own so little. They can and they do take the risks which have to be taken if the Establishment is to be challenged. Thus it can be seen that this old conflict between youth and their elders, which has existed for centuries, is nothing to worry about, in fact it is desirable.

THE NEW CONFLICT

The conflict which needs explanation and about which we are rightly concerned is a new development. This appeared on the horizon only in the past decade and has affected most of the countries in the Western Hemisphere. This conflict is not related only to the youth of an oppressed minority where it would be easily understandable, but involves a large number of young people from relatively affluent families. This conflict first became apparent in the uprisings at Berkeley, California, and since then has manifested itself in other areas in the world.

On listening to the demands and the protests of the young the reaction of the older generation is not only that of anger and disagreement but also of complete incomprehension, as if the two groups are speaking two different languages. This conflict cannot be explained simply by such concepts as generation gap or adolescent rebellion.

An Explanation

It is suggested that if we are perplexed by the behavior of the young we can reach an understanding of their present-day behavior by looking at what happened to them in their formative years. If one assumes that a child is born without any moral, social or ethical values, then one must assume that the attitudes he displays as an adolescent must have been acquired in his early years. If one agrees that home and school environments are the molds which give shape to a generation, then logically one place to look for an answer as to why the young believe what they believe and do what they do is to find out what happened to them in their homes and schools during their formative years. This traditional psychiatric approach of going back into the past to explain what appears unexplainable from the present perspective is applied here, in the hope that it will add to our understanding. This is not to deny that there are many factors in the present, such as the Vietnam War, social injustices, and at times the mishandling of reasonable requests from students, which could explain certain events. There is, however, a feeling shared by many observers of the present scene, that there is something uniquely and radically different, nowadays, in the attitude of the young toward authority. This authority may be represented by a police officer, the dean of a university, the mayor of a city, or the President of the United States. It is suggested here that this changed attitude toward authority is the central determining factor which explains many actions of the young today. The young people feel that whoever represents authority owes them an explanation for all his actions. The age, experience and position of the person in authority are no substitute and are no guarantee against mistakes or immoral decisions.

To trace the origin of this posture toward authority one should discover what attitudes were inculcated in today's youth during their childhood.

There is a great deal of evidence to show that child-rearing habits, classroom discipline and the role of the teacher were radically altered after World War II. New theories emerged about how children should be raised. In the past, parents generally brought up their children in very much the same way as they themselves could remember having been brought up.

In the past 25 years the rapid rate of technological advance with its accompanying socioeconomic change has affected every part of the fabric of our society. The mass instant communication, the unprecedented affluence and, most important, the explosion of knowledge have created a situation where a great deal of what a father learned in school is out of date when his son arrives at school. This has made parents believe that their own experiences no longer provide relevant guidelines for them to use in bringing up their children. With grandparents in most cases out of the picture the parents began to look to the experts to find out "what to do when Johnny refuses to eat." The need for this information coincided with the appearance of Dr. Spock's book, the child guidance clinics, magazines for parents and the child psychiatrists. In advice given by the professionals, the emphasis was changed from obedience to autonomy. We must explain to the child before we expect obedience. We must also admit when we are wrong. Relationships with adults should be less formal and more flexible. This resulted in a changed attitude toward authority, both at home and at school. Little Johnny was telling his father that he was wrong and schoolteachers were being called by their first names.

This changed attitude toward authority, this encouragement of individual expression as opposed to mere obedience, this new wave of liberalism both at home and at school meant that children were not being molded in the same way as previous generations had been. In fact, without recognizing it, without making a conscious decision, we were producing a different kind of person. These individuals were brought up to question rather than to obey, to think for themselves rather than to follow, and to think that elders are not necessarily right. Initiative was at least as important as experience and, in fact, the latter may only be a hindrance. We told them to take nothing for granted. Everything was open to question, from God to basic sexual morals. Without recognizing it we changed our child-rearing habits and our school discipline and have thus produced a generation with radically different expectations and attitudes. However, at the same time we did not prepare ourselves or our institutions to receive and accommodate this new breed.

Why the Conflict

We expected these children to grow up into young adults and behave in a manner similar to that of any young generation of former years. We hoped they would follow Harold Coffin's advice that there is nothing like becoming established to cure one's dissatisfaction with the Establishment. We expected that there would be the usual conflict arising out of the so-called generation gap, but this conflict we are witnessing is not simply of differences between young and old. This conflict exists because we shaped these young adults differently, with the result that they have radically different expectations and attitudes, especially in relation to authority and regulations. They want to know why they must go into the army, why they must take examinations. They want to question everything before accepting anything, from God to the constitution of their own country, just as we taught them to do. The riots, the protests, the questioning, the challenging are the force and the noise of a round peg trying to fit into a square hole. If we had had the foresight we would have prepared ourselves and our institutions to receive this new breed that we produced. If we have the understanding we will make the necessary changes required to accommodate this new generation. Changes should not necessarily have to wait for confrontations. We should move away from the question of right and wrong. It is not useful to discuss whether we were wise to bring up our children as we did. The conflict is due to the fact that we brought about changes on one end without preparing ourselves to receive the consequences on the other. One simply cannot change the shape and design of the parts and expect that they will fit into the old structure. If such a happening had taken place in the automobile industry and if one had received parts which simply did not fit into the old structure, one would return the parts and ask for replacements that would fit. It would be an easy solution if we could do the same with our youth—return them to the factory, say that we made a mistake and ask for the necessary alterations. For better or worse, and I, for one, believe for the better, we have produced a generation that is radically different from any previous generation. This generation will change our institutions and the structure of our society.

The Future

The question is: "Are we going to continue to be amazed and shocked by the behavior of the youth whose attitudes and ethics we have been responsible for shaping, or are we going to help our institutions to adjust so that this new generation can be absorbed?" The answer to this question will determine whether we will continue to have the riots and the destruction which have taken place in the past few years.

REFERENCES

Erikson, E. H., Ed. (1963): *Youth: Change and Challenge.* Basic Books, New York.

Jencks, C., and Riesman, D. (1968): *The Academic Revolution.* Doubleday & Co., New York.

Keniston, K. (1968): *Young Radicals.* Harcourt, Brace & World Inc., New York.

Lipset, S. M., and Wolin, S. S. (1965): *The Berkeley Student Revolt.* Anchor Books, New York.

Mead, M. (1928): *Coming of Age in Samoa.* William Morrow & Co., Inc., New York.

Chapter 13

EVOLVING PERSPECTIVES ON DRUG USE BY YOUTH

John R. Unwin

> Up from the pastures of boredom
> out from the sea of discontent
> they come in packs like hungry hounds
> the seekers of the dark enchantment.
>
> McKuen 1967

No book, conference, symposium, panel, prayer—nothing dedicated to contemporary youth seems complete or relevant without due reference to the use and misuse of psychoactive drugs. This topic, with its guaranteed paradoxes and controversies, may have been manna from heaven for the communications media, but for those who work with youth (tranquil, troubled or troublesome) the phenomenon has more the qualities of a plague. One can envy Winston Churchill, reporting in 1898, when he was able "to pass with relief from the tossing sea of Cause and Theory to the firm ground of Result and Fact." Such an opportunity continues to elude those who contemplate and confront the youth "drug scene"; to most it remains essentially "a riddle wrapped in a mystery inside an enigma" (again the phrase is Churchill's).

It has become increasingly clear that a significant aspect of this difficulty is the rather stubborn and narrow focus on *youth* and its preferred drugs (especially the cannabis products). A broader perspective is imperative if we are to construct effective and appropriate social responses to the problem; such a perspective is embodied in the mandate of the current Canadian Federal Commission of Inquiry into the Non-Medical Use of Drugs (the so-called LeDain Commission, 1970). This Commission has been required to study, in the broadest possible medical, sociologic and philosophic terms the use and misuse *not* of marijuana, *not* of drugs by youth, but of all psychoactive drugs by the total Canadian population. The following figures may help widen our perspective: in metropolitan Toronto 1,369,000 prescriptions are issued yearly for mood-modifying drugs. This number exceeds the adult population of that area, where on any given day one person in every seven is under the influence of legally prescribed tranquilizers, stimulants, etc. (*Medical Post,* 1970). This survey indicates that mood-modifying drugs account for 24 percent of all medical prescriptions; over one half of such drugs prescribed in hospitals are issued through nonpsychiatric clinics. Note that the above figures relate only to legitimate prescriptions; they do not include narcotics, "over-the-counter" preparations, or any illicit drugs. Another survey, conducted by the Canadian Medical Association (Canad. Med. Assoc., 1971) on "the current use of stimulants and sedatives in [Canadian] medicine," found that during the chosen survey week 32.9 percent of all prescriptions issued were for mood-modifying drugs; of these, 35.5 percent were for minor tranquilizers, 20.3 percent for barbiturates, 6.9 percent for amphetamines and amphetamine-like drugs. "More than half of all mood-modifying Rx's were of a repeat nature, varying from 48 percent for non-barbiturate (sedatives) to 64 percent for amphetamines." Recent Federal statistics suggest that 20 to 25 percent of Canadian adults are prescribed an amphetamine or barbiturate each year. H. David Archibald, executive director of Ontario's Addiction Research Foundation, estimates that about 23 percent of the adult population of Ontario consume the equivalent of 7 ounces or more of whisky [about 3 ounces of alcohol] each day (*Montreal Star,* Jan. 1971).

ADULT PRACTICES AND ATTITUDES

Further details about our *over*-18 North American population may set youth practices in a wider and more valid context. What of illicit drug use by adults? A 1967–68 study (Manheimer et al., 1969) of a representative sample of the over-18 population of San Francisco indicated that 13 percent had used marijuana and 3 percent LSD. During the 1969 hearings of the LeDain Commission, a journalist testified in Vancouver that the 44 reporters on two newspapers of that city were regular marijuana smokers. In 1971 a policeman, formerly a youth squad member, admitted in Montreal to the illegal possession of hashish (*Montreal star,* June 1971). Other examples of Canadian adult illicit drug use are readily available (though much of the evidence so far has been mainly anecdotal) (LeDain Commission, 1970; Ruddy, 1969). There is serious concern in the United States about the spread of drug use in the automobile and other industries (*Montreal Gazette,* April 1970; Amer. Soc. Health Assoc., 1970) and among junior business executives (*Montreal Star,* Sept. 1970) Pilots of the U.S. Strategic Air Command have been found in possession of marijuana and other drugs (*Montreal Star,* Aug. 1970) and the drug practices of other U.S. militzary personnel on active duty (particularly in Vietnam) have been well publicized and studied (Black et al., 1970;

Colbach, 1971). The incidence of heroin dependence, which was sensationally exaggerated initially, but is nonetheless significant, among GIs due for discharge from Vietnam threatens serious public health problems for North America—not the least of which could be the reintroduction of malaria to this continent. Carriers, infected in Vietnam, could spread the disease through blood donations and through the communal use of nonsterile needles and syringes within the heroin and methamphetamine subcultures.

Add to the above cursory overview the volume of "over-the-counter" mood-modifying drugs used (freely available without prescription, and "pushed" day and night through the communications media, *ad nauseam* and *ad infinitum*) and it becomes obvious that, in the area of the misuse of psychoactive drugs, the much-flaunted "generation gap" has been successfully bridged! Our adult population needs to moderate considerably its wildly excessive use of contemporary youth as projection and displacement targets (i.e., scapegoats); our entire population must realize that we live in a "drug culture" (Andrew Malcolm's "chemophilic society" [1971, p. 351]) wherein, increasingly, a significant segment of our people exhibits a cavalier attitude towards the "self-prescription" of a wide variety of psychoactive substances.

ADULTS AS MODELS FOR YOUTH

It may seem naive to suggest that during the past 5 years or so, while youth presented itself as dissident and alienated, vociferously challenging and allegedly rejecting conventional parental values and ethics, nevertheless adults (and particularly parents) were acting as identification figures, at least in the area of drug use. A study in 1953 (Straus and Bacon, 1953) had indicated how strongly then, parental attitudes and practices influenced their offspring's drug (alcohol) habits—but the youth of the 1950's (the so-called "cool" or "quiet" generation) fitted nicely into our understanding of adolescent psychologic and sociologic development and it was minimal wisdom for professionals to appreciate that parents, albeit by their practices rather than their pronouncements, unwittingly served as value- and attitude-models for their children. But what about the parents of the dissident youth of the 1960's? It is only recently, in fact since 1970, that reliable research has indicated just how much parental drug habits are influencing youth. A survey in two Niagara (Ontario) counties (Smart et al., 1970A) showed such a significant relationship between parental (particularly maternal) use of mood-modifying drugs and high-school student use of illicit drugs that the researchers concluded: "Unless the present results are misread, any substantial reduction in adolescent drug use or abuse will occur only after a reduction in parental drug use." Thus, mothers who used tranquilizers daily were three times as likely to have children using cannabis, LSD or solvents than mothers who did not use tranquilizers. Furthermore, mothers using tranquilizers daily were five times as likely to have children using stimulants and seven times as likely to have offspring using tranquilizers and barbiturates. A subsequent study in Toronto (Smart et. al., 1970B) confirmed these findings and concluded that "education methods will have to involve parents to a much greater extent than has been done so far. ... *Current adolescent drug use has its roots in the larger society and in aspects of adult behavior.* (italics mine] Efforts to concentrate drug abuse prevention and control on young persons will probably be ineffective." (These findings are not uniquely Canadian—speaking before a U.S. Senate subcommittee in July 1971, Dr. Donald Louria reported evidence of similar parental influence in a United States study conducted within the preceding year.)

CURRENT USE OF DRUGS BY YOUTH

In Toronto high schools, in the 2 years between 1968 and 1970, there was a virtual tripling in the use, for example, of marijuana and LSD (Smart et al., 1970B) despite the activities of law-enforcement agencies and despite special education programs in the schools. The increase involved both number of users and frequency of use, with a marked trend towards multiple-drug use (Dr. Lionel Solursh's "chemical promiscuity"). In these 2 years, the percentage of students using cannabis products rose from 6.7 to 18.3 percent, LSD from 2.6 to 8.5 percent and such opiates as morphine (not necessarily illicitly) and heroin from 1.9 to 4 percent. Smart and Fejer (1971) comment that "perhaps family therapy rather than individual or group therapy is required. It also seems evident that the target population for drug education should not be students but entire families."

The projected trend? "At the present rate of increase it would take only four years until marijuana is used by more students than is alcohol and less than six years until everyone is using marijuana. Methods for preventing this development have not yet been found" (Smart et al., 1970B). Based on previous surveys using essentially the same methodology as the above study, it seems reasonable to assume that the Toronto developments will be replicated by findings on students in Montreal and Halifax (Smart and Fejer, 1971).

With regard to university students, a recent nation-wide survey in the United States (Dep't. of Soc. Relations, Johns Hopkins Univ., 1970) indicates that some 31 percent of the respondents were using marijuana once every week or two during the period of the survey. Previous experience (LeDain Commission, 1970; Unwin, 1969, 1970: *McGill News,* March 1969) suggests that average U.S. figures will be approximated in Canadian universities within 12 to 18 months. Moving back towards (young) adult illicit drug use, it is striking that in recent surveys of university students by faculty, the highest incidence figures tend increasingly to be found in the medical faculties. Thus, at McGill University, 40 percent of the medical students in 1969 admitted to cannabis use within the preceding 6 months (Caron). A 1970 comparative study of the final-year medical student classes at the University of Toronto and at U.C.L.A. in California (Solursh et al., 1971) revealed: cannabis use at least once: U. of T. 43 percent, U.C.L.A. 73 percent; current cannabis use once or more per month: U. of T. 13 percent, U.C.L.A. 41 percent. Lipp, Benson and Taintor (1971) in 1970 received responses from 1063 medical students at four widely-separated medical schools in the United States to the effect that 50 percent had used marijuana at least once in the past, while 30 percent admitted current use. The range for the four schools, for at least one experience with cannabis, was from 17 percent at one school to 70 percent at another. Another faculty which tends to give high figures is law: 73 percent of U.C.L.A. law students (Lipp et al., 1971), and 27 percent of McGill University law students (Caron) have used cannabis at least once.

What do these figures about our medical and law students indicate—especially in view of the fact that they of all students should be well informed about the medical and legal consequences of illicit use of drugs? Are they criminals? (They are by law, though surely not by common sense.) What percentage will later become dependent on opiates? Certainly their future influence in society will mold public and legislative opinions on the drug issue. Are their attitudes towards cannabis more reasonable than those of many members of the professions they are about to join? Lipp, Benson and Taintor conclude that "there is a vast gulf between the position of the medical profession and the position of the medical student"

(Lipp et al., 1971). During another presentation of his findings (*Medical Post,* Nov. 1970), Dr. Lipp noted that "the respondents, whether they smoke marijuana or not, regard it as a relatively harmless agent that should be made more widely available without penalties." In a breakdown of the various faculties, another study (Mizner et al., 1970) found the highest incidence of amphetamine use among students of medicine and nursing. As a cautionary note, one must weigh carefully the findings of a Tuft's University group (*The Horner Newsletter,* April 1970 who compared 45 physicians (judged 20 years previously, as sophomores, to be psychologically healthy) with 90 controls. The 45 physicians took more mood-modifying drugs than the controls (although the two groups broke even for alcohol and tobacco use). Self-medication with drugs or alcohol was the cause of one third of the total time spent as patients in hospitals by these doctors. The conclusion of the Tuft's team, reinforcing what health professionals know but do not pass onto their students, is that they represent a particularly high-risk population for drug dependence (Modlin and Montes, 1964).

The various figures quoted above for the different categories of students in high school and university will be criticized (probably with some justification) by users as being unduly conservative. But the studies from which they are derived remain, on the whole, islands of reasonable reliability in a sea of impressionistic reports, such as the World Health Organization estimate of more than 200 million regular cannabis users throughout the world (*Canadian Doctor,* 1971) or the frequently quoted estimates of from 12 million to 20 million regular cannabis users in the United States. It does seem reasonable, however, to assume that the use of cannabis is now pandemic (at least in industrial and post-industrial nations); the circumstances of its distribution, availability and use bear all the hallmarks of the (alcohol) Prohibition Era in the United

States, including the inefficacy and frequent destructiveness of the pertinent laws. Anticipated and necessary changes in Canadian laws will presumably await the Final Report of the LeDain Commission (due in late 1971); in its Interim Report (1970) this Commission recommended as a matter of some urgency that simple possession of *any* psychoactive drug should no longer be punishable by imprisonment—a recommendation which became Canadian Medical Association policy in June 1971.

THE FORGOTTEN DRUG

The greatest amount of study, concern and controversy has centered on the use of cannabis products by youth. Yet which *is* the psychoactive substance most commonly involved in illegal use and legal misuse by youth? *Alcohol* —a drug inviting both psychologic and physical dependence (that is, "addiction"); a drug which can be associated with serious physical and psychiatric illness (acute and chronic), and which even in so-called "social" use can be a menace to society. Drinken drivers killed over 2500 persons in Canada in 1969; very high blood alcohol concentrations are found in more than 50 percent of persons responsible for fatal automobile accidents (Campbell, 1969, 1971), and one study (Campbell, 1971) notes specifically that "some of our [Canadian] underage drivers are very seriously involved with alcohol." (The relationship of drugs other than alcohol to highway accidents is far less clear [Waller, 1971].)

The Toronto 2-year follow-up study (Smart et al., 1970B) notes: "Alcohol, by far the most widely used drug, is now [in 1970] used by approximately one-third more [high-school] students than in 1968." Further, "heavy" alcohol users increased among these students by 41 percent in the 2 years. (The sharpest rise in alcohol use was among seventh-grade students.) It is incredible that when these various youth drug surveys are reported, the greatest concern and indignation centers around the cannabis figures (despite the fact that, according to current knowledge and judgment, cannabis is among the least potentially harmful drugs in popular use); virtually no public or professional attention or concern is paid to the figures for alcohol use in these same surveys, even though the alcohol figures more often than not exceed by far those of all the other drugs combined. Yet Jellineck, a leading authority on alcoholism, has warned that one third of those who become alcoholics in the United States have their initial drinking experiences between the ages of 14 and 18 years and show the prodromal signs of alcohol dependence between the ages of 18 and 21 (Alcohol Studies Guide, 1968).

DANGEROUS OR HARMLESS?

I have, in previous publications (Unwin, 1969, 1970, 1968), reviewed the various drugs in popular use among youth—their nature, incidence, mode of use, effects, hazards, social consequences and legal implications— and the Interim Report of the LeDain Commission (1970) provides an excellent concise overview of the Canadian picture. Compact, reliable guides for the management of drug crises are available (Mackenzie and Garell, 1971; Schoichet and Solursh, 1969), and the formidable task of keeping *au courant* with the continually changing youth drug scene, with its cornucopia of substances, is considerably simplified by a free subscription to the reliable, brief and eminently readable STASH *Capsules* produced by the Students Association for the Study of Hallucinogens, Inc. These *Capsules* (newsletters) are more liable to be experienced as credible by youth than most of the other material available.

As adequate descriptive and consultative material is available, I will avoid the detailed discussion of specific drugs and suggest instead a type of framework within which all psychoactive substances can be placed in a perspective which can be comprehensible to the population-at-risk (which, as we have seen, knows no age boundaries). To speak of any drug as being simply "harmful" or "harmless" is misleading and confusing; obviously there is virtually no substance which cannot be introduced into the body in some form or concentration, or by some route, without causing serious physical and psychiatric illness (and, in fact, even death). And one includes here air and water (perhaps especially air and water in view of the current environmental crisis!). It would seem to be more appropriate and clarifying to speak of the *relative potential* for harm of a given substance (relative, that is, to other drugs). Furthermore, each substance's potential for harm should be rated (say, on a five-point scale) separately for physical health, mental health, social consequences (and advisedly, legal consequences, given the current absurdity of our laws). Using such a composite weighting (but ignoring the illogicality of the drug laws) it would seem reasonable to construct a hierarchy of drugs, beginning with those with the greatest composite potential for harm. Such an abbreviated hierarchy might be:

1. The solvents and stimulants (including cocaine)
2. The depressants: hypnotics, true narcotics, alcohol, minor tranquilizers, certain "over-the-counter" preparations
3. The "psychedelics": LSD, mescaline, psilocybin, DMT, etc.
4. Cannabis products: marijuana and hashish

Placing cannabis at the bottom of this abbreviated list does *not* imply that it is "harmless" but that, in the light of current knowledge (Amer. J. Psychiat., 1971), it has relatively less potential for harm to the average person and to society than the other substances listed. Let me repeat, there is no "harmless" psychoactive drug at present in known use. And there is likely to be little disagreement that allowing the younger adolescent free, unsupervised access to *any* intoxicant (including alcohol) must be considered unacceptably hazardous during such a critical phase of the development of his physical, psychologic, social and intellectual capacities.

THE HIDDEN AGENDA

Such attempts at organization and perspective as the above hierarchy do not, unfortunately, seem to lessen the confusion and controversy as much as one might hope— and the center of the storm is inevitably cannabis. In the "Review and Position Paper" of the Canadian Medical Association Brief to the LeDain Commission (Unwin, 1969) I have attempted to identify and analyze the factors which have prevented (and to this day continue to obstruct) reasonable consensus on social responses and policies towards this substance. Of the various factors identified, it seems to me that the most crucial now is the *symbolic significance* which marijuana (and hashish) has attained. To quote, "marijuana use has become a symbol upon which contemporary society has projected its anxieties, desires, or indignations. . . . It seems almost impossible to find a middle ground from which to approach the many controversial issues involved, and polarisation of opinion is more common than detached scientific assessment. Attitudes towards marijuana reflect many of the central dilemmas of a society in perennial rapid transition. To some, marijuana use seems to represent all that is disturbed and disturbing about (the more visible segments of) contemporary youth—the protestors, 'hippies,' student activists, educational and social drop-outs, a 'permissive' society, etc. To others it evokes other concerns—the apparent arbitrariness of overcentralised, distant authority, the impersonality of administrative decision-making, the relative obsolescence of tradition, inconsistencies in the formulation and enforcement of laws, and the diminishing reliability and relevance of conventional wisdom and values in the face of burgeoning technology" (Unwin 1969).

It has become glaringly clear that a simple, "damn the torpedoes" approach to the resolution of such a complex, emotionally charged (and therefore prejudiced) issue will be both inefficacious and disruptive. A Past-President of the Canadian Psychiatric Association asserted in 1970 that "authority for decision-making on social conduct rests with the more experienced and learned, that is, with sapiential authority. The policy of unbalanced permissiveness in this century is proving untimely and premature and is leading to anarchic chaos. A greater degree of sapiential authority needs to be demonstrated and exerted today—specifically, for example, with regard to the drug problem and its associated wave of socio-cultural ferment" (Yonge, 1970). Even if one could accept such a postulate in toto, the bewildering challenge remains as to how to identify and accredit such "sapiential authority." Already in previous publications it has been demonstrated (Unwin, 1969, 1970) how authorities with impeccable credentials have offered mutually contradictory opinions and approaches to the same information or problem—and more recent examples abound. Thus, another Past-President of the Canadian Psychiatric Association recommended (also in 1970) that "simple possession of a psychedelic drug and cannabis products . . . should not be punishable by law" (Medical Action for Mental Health, 1970)—an opinion at variance with that of the other Past-President quoted (Yonge, 1970). Which is the "sapiential authority"? From the same information in the National Institute of Mental Health report to the U.S. Congress in January 1971 (*Amer. J. Psychiat.,* 1971), the U.S. Department of Defense deduced that cannabis products were definitely harmful, while the U.S. Department of Health, Education and Welfare concluded that no conclusions were possible as to the harmfulness or harmlessness of the substance. While the Ontario Medical Association (*Ont. Med. Review,* July 1971) has recommended removal of simple possession of marijuana from the Criminal Code of Canada, and the Canadian Medical Association has recommended the abolition of prison sentences for simple possession of all psychoactive drugs (including cannabis, narcotics, LSD, etc.) (Canad Med. Assoc., 1971), the Government of the Province of Saskatchewan (*Montreal Star,* Nov. 1970) has indicated its strong opposition to any easing of Canadian drug laws. The noted anthropologist Dr. Margaret Mead recommended to a U.S. Senate subcommittee (*Montreal Gazette,* Oct. 1969) that not only should marijuana be legalized in the United States, but that it should probably be made available for use at age 16. President Nixon, on the other hand, has stated that, even should his own appointed commission on marijuana so recommend, he would not agree to legalization of the substance. Many other examples of the difficulty in objectively and dispassionately identifying "sapiential authority" are available, but the exercise is already unduly tedious and too many opinions tendentious.

Of the many multidetermined issues for which the cannabis controversy has become a symbol and rallying-flag, one which is preeminent is the attempt of contemporary society and its institutions to adapt appropriately to continual rapid change. The impact of technology and of the changes it is already enforcing on social structures and values has been persuasively portrayed by Toffler in his book *Future Shock* (Toffler, 1970). Within our own professional activities with youth, and in the youth-rearing and care-taking institutions of society, the aim has been to help youth adapt to the "average expectable environment." What anticipatory adjustments do we (and will we continuously) need in an evolving society in which the definition and parameters of the "average" are becoming increasingly blurred and in which events seem to be less and less "expectable"? The essence of the matter is stated by Kahn and Wiener of the Hudson Institute (Kahn and Wiener, 1968): "The pace with which such changes are taking place has reduced the reliability of practical experience as a guide to public policy and has diminished the usefulness of practical experience in dealing with social problems. . . . Policy-makers in many fields, given so much new information to assimilate, so many new variables to assess, and so little experience directly relevant to the new problems, can no longer be as confident of the applicability of traditional wisdom and can no longer rely as much on the intuitively derived judgements that once seemed so adequate to resolve issues and to achieve fairly well-understood social goals." Jean-Jacques Servan Schreiber (Servan-Schreiber, 1968) underlines the point: "A century ago there was time for reflection, time for the traditional information system to bring new information to the decision-makers before undesirable applications took place, but the traditional system is now inadequate. If we continue to rely on it, we will be making our decisions more and more by chance."

What to do, in view of the foregoing? Toffler (1970) suggests a stratagem which will be more and more commonly used in the future to tackle new, unconventional social problems: the temporary task force. We do in fact have such groups in existence at the present time—the LeDain Commission in Canada, presidential commissions in the United States. And rather than the individual judgment of one consultant we have in these commissions the amalgamated judgment, experience and wisdom of members who surely manifest *collective* "sapiential authority"—by virtue of their individual credentials, their eminence in their fields of endeavor, and by virtue of the action of governments in instituting such commissions. Can we agree that such groups are more likely than any other device to reach reasonable (not infallible) approaches towards a resolution of the drug problem? Can we persuade governments, and our society, that action on the findings and recommendations of these commissions is a matter of urgent priority—given the irony that there have been, since the beginning of this century, at least five previous similar official commissions throughout the English-speaking world whose findings, on cannabis, for example, have been remarkably similar, but on whose recommendations governments have repeatedly failed to act in any significant manner. We cannot afford to await the Second Coming.

REFERENCES

Alcohol Studies Guide (1968): Addiction Research Foundation and Ontario Department of Education, Toronto, p. 27.

Black, S., Owens, K. L., and Wolff, R. P. (1970): Patterns of drug use: a study of 5,482 subjects, Amer. J. Psychiat. 127: 62–65.

Campbell, E. (1969): Alcohol involvement in fatal motor vehicle accidents. Mod. Med. Canad. 24: 35–42.

Campbell, E. (1971): Alcohol involvement in fatal motor vehicle accidents 1966–1969. Mod. Med. Canad. 26:7–10.

Caron, P. (1970): Personal communication.

Colbach, E. (1971): Marijuana use by G.Is. in Viet Nam. Amer. J. Psychiat. 218:204–207.

Drug Abuse in Industry (1970): American Social Health Association, New York.

Final Brief of the Canadian Medical Association to the Commission of Inquiry into the Non-Medical Use of Drugs, Canadian Medical Association, Ottawa, 1971.

Heavy use of mood modifers revealed in Toronto (1970). Med. Post 6:17, June 16.

Interim Report of the Commission of Inquiry into the Non-Medical Use of Drugs (1970). Queen's Printer, Ottawa. (Report of Le Dain Commission).

Kahn, H., and Wiener, A. J. (1968): *The Year 2000*. Macmillan Co., New York.

Lipp, M. R., Benson, S. S., and Taintor, Z. (1971): Marijuana use by medical students. Amer. J. Psychiat. 128:207–212.

Mackenzie, R. G., and Garell, D. C. (1971): Practical approaches to management of drug abuse. Adolescent Medicine Newsletter 6:8–14.

Malcolm, A. I. (1971): *The Pursuit of Intoxication.* Addiction Research Foundation of Ontario, Toronto.

Manheimer, D. I., Mellinger, G. D., and Balter, M. B. (1969): Marijuana among urban adults. Science 166:1544-1547.

Marijuana examined (1971). Canadian Doctor 37: 21–23.

Marijuana and health: a report to the Congress (1971). Amer. J. Psychiat. 128:189–193.

McGill News (Montreal) 50: 3, March 1969.

McKuen, R. (1967): The lovers. In: *Listen to the Warm.* Random House, New York.

Medical Action for Mental Health: Problems of Childhood and Youth (1970). Proceedings of national conference, Canadian Medical Association, Ottawa, p. 12, Recommendation XXI.

Mizner, G. L., Barter, J. T. and Werme, P. H. (1970): Patterns to drug use among college students: a preliminary report. Amer. J. Psychiat. 127: 15–24.

Modlin, H. C. and Montes, A. (1964): Narcotics addiction in physicians. Amer. J. Psychiat. 121:358–365.

Montreal Gazette, October 28, 1969, p. 5.; also personal communication.

Montreal Gazette, April 22, 1970.

Montreal Star, August 19, 1970, p. 73.

Montreal Star, September 3, 1970, p. 23.

Montreal Star, November 14, 1970, p. 9.

Montreal Star, January 2, 1971, p. 21.

Montreal Star, June 17, 1971.

Ontario Medical Review, July 1971, pp. 354–355.

Ruddy, J. (1969): Some of the best people smoke pot. MacLean's Magazine, 82(1): 35–40, January.

Servan-Schreiber, J.-J. (1968): *The American Challenge.* Atheneum, New York.

Schoichet, R. and Solursh, L. (1969): Treatment of the hallucinogenic drug crisis. Appl. Ther. 11: 283–286.

Smart, R. G., Fejer, D., and Alexander, E. (1970A): *Drug Use among High School Students and Their Parents in Lincoln and Welland Counties.* Addiction Research Foundation, Toronto.

Smart, R. G., Fejer, D., and White, J. (1970B): *The Extent of Drug Use in Metropolitan Toronto Schools: a Study of Changes from 1968 to 1970.* Addiction Research Foundation, Toronto.

Smart, R. G., and Fejer, D. (1971): Recent trends in illicit drug use among adolescents. Canada's Mental Health, Supplement No. 68.

Solursh, L. P., Weinstock, S. M., Saunders, C. S., and Ungerleider, J. T. (1971): Attitudes of medical students to cannabis. J.A.M.A. (in press for September).

STASH Capsules, The Student Association for the Study of Hallucinogens, Inc., 638 Pleasant Street, Beloit, Wisconsin 53511.

Straus, R. and Bacon, S. D. (1953): *Drinking In College*. Yale University Press, New Haven.

Study of Life Styles and Campus Communities, Preliminary report (1970). Department of Social Relations, Johns Hopkins University, Baltimore.

Study shows doctors use more mood-altering drugs (1970). The Horner Newsletter, Vol. 7, No. 4 April 6.

Toffler, A. (1970): *Future Shock*. Random House, New York.

Unwin, J. R. (1968): Illicit drug use among Canadian youth. Canad. Med. Assoc. J. 98:402–407 and 449–454.

Unwin, J. R. (1969): Non-medical use of drugs with particular reference to youth. Review and Position Paper prepared as integral part of the Canadian Medical Association Interim Brief to the Commission of Inquiry into the Non-Medical Use of Drugs. Canad. Med. Assoc. J. 101:804–820.

Unwin, J. R. (1970): Contemporary misuse of psychoactive drugs by youth. In: *The World Biennial of Psychiatry and Psychotherapy,* Vol. 1, S. Arieti, Ed. Basic Books, New York, pp. 426–459.

Waller, J. A. (1971): Drugs and highway crashes. J.A.M.A. 215:1477-1482.

World medical law meeting ranges from malpractice to marijuana in med-school (1970). Medical Post 6:18–19, November 3.

Yonge, K. A. (1970): Looking with the third eye. Canad. Psychiat. Assoc. J. 15:413–422.

Chapter 14

GROUPS FOR YOUTH
IN THE EVERYDAY WORLD

Beryce W. MacLennan

In this chapter, interventions are discussed which build opportunities for psychotherapy and self-development into the everyday life of the adolescent. These approaches emphasize the individual's desires, goals, and strengths rather than his failures and inadequacies. Problems are viewed as normal events to be tackled and resolved. Groups which form part of the ordinary life of the adolescent are utilized as media for change.

Whether these interventions are defined as psychotherapy, self-development, or merely as assisting individuals to cope more adequately in some aspect of daily living, they are concerned with the achievement of changes in the individual's psychic structure and functioning. They aim to assist a youth to feel more satisfied with and in himself, develop more harmonious relationships with his environment, and mobilize himself to best advantage. Change is achieved when the individual gains a new perspective on himself and his world. He may feel differently about himself and learn new skills in expressing himself and coping with his world through new experiences or through increased understanding of himself and his environment. Efforts to change are geared to what changes are needed and can be planned at a variety of levels and with many different methods. The method will depend both on goals and the particular theory of change held by the therapist. Goals can be very limited or aimed at basic alterations in the personality. They can be directed *primarily toward giving information* about problems and alternatives for action, toward the *resolution of specific problems* or toward *over-all changes in self-concept and self-management* (MacLennan, 1968, and MacLennan and Felsenfeld, 1970). Groups can be *conducted at a guidance level* which explores feelings, problems, and alternatives. They can *utilize psychoanalytic techniques* which stimulate intensive emotional transactions, which are then analyzed and understood. They can rework and reinforce certain kinds of behavior, can concentrate on exercises which sensitize members to become more aware of their physical and emotional reactions, or can focus on assisting individuals to live more actively in the present.

However, all permanent intrapsychic change is made in and by the individual and cannot be achieved against his will. No change will occur unless the forces within him are on balance in favor of making change. At some level, the patient must want to mobilize himself in a positive direction. But, when an individual seeks or is sent for psychotherapy, he is immediately confronted with the recognition that there is something which is not satisfactory about himself and his functioning, that he is in some way deviant, and that he is not adequate to make the necessary changes on his own. He must seek help from an expert and place himself in a dependent position. At a minimal level, he must accept the authority of the therapist or the therapeutic agent. He must agree to expose himself and to surrender some control over himself (MacLennan, 1968).

Because adolescence is the period of transition from childhood to adult life and the individual must make many changes, this posture can be particularly hard for the teenager. During this time, the process of maturation is accelerated; and youth must create an adult identity, socially, sexually, and vocationally. Boys and girls become more urgently aware of their sexual desires and wish to test out and experience sexual activity. They struggle to become self-reliant, to create a way of life for themselves, and to gain confidence in themselves as individuals. Curiosity and experimentation with new ways are natural and an important part of growing up. Temporary rejection of surrounding adults and their values can be seen as functional in these efforts. Breaking away from reliance on the family is an essential part of the process. However, this abandonment of the security of the home and of the familiar and often comfortable dependence on childhood authorities is difficult. When parents and other adults resist the movement toward independence and refuse to accept teenagers as fully respected fellow human beings, they make the struggle more intense. The youth are often beset by self-doubt and uncertainty. Their confidence wanes, and they become excessively dependent, depressed, and despairing, or over-determinedly defiant. Their need to feel confident, competent, and self-reliant is often so great that the patient position is strongly resisted and, indeed, can be viewed as going against the life force of the individual and, consequently, inappropriate for this age (MacLennan 1968).

Moreover, it has also become clear that often when an individual is given a particular reputation, stereotyped into a negative role, and thus stigmatized by the community, both the organizational structures and the individual's own feelings about himself conspire to make him live out the role (Goffman, 1963). For instance, when an individual is called mentally ill or delinquent, people start relating differently to him. They expect him to be queer, dangerous, or irresponsible; and he is set apart and barred from many opportunities. In his anger and despair, he may well accept the role, cease to struggle against the pressures and behave defiantly in the ways which are expected of him.

In recognition of this, attempts have been made over the last few years to structure the therapeutic situation differently so that the relationship between the individual and the change agent is a less threatening one, and the intervention utilizes the constructive needs and desires of the youth. In such approaches, the strengths and achievements of the individual are emphasized and problems are considered as blocks to the attainment of the youth's aspirations (MacLennan, 1968 MacLennan and Felsenfeld, 1970).

The need for change is not presented as a special and abnormal event but rather as a normal aspect and an integral part of all living. In this framework, treatment might preferably be called assistance in personal development rather than therapy. Such interventions take place in normal settings, such as schools, colleges, youth residences, recreational clubs, employment counseling agencies, churches, youth leadership and job training programs, research programs, and on the job itself. The youth do not see themselves as patients but as students, members, research informants, colleagues, co-leaders, participants, helpers, trainees, or individuals seeking assistance in making plans for normal living.

Groups are emphasized because they dilute the tensions between the adult and the youth and because of the normal tendency of teenagers to turn for support to their peers. Groups are also the medium of choice because they provide natural opportunities for interaction and reality testing.

The group selected as the vehicle of change is one to

which the individual normally belongs in his daily life: a class, a club, a planning group, a work team; and the therapists are also teachers, recreation leaders, residence directors, research workers, work supervisors, trainers. Their function as change agents is built-in as one aspect of a non-therapeutic role. Aims may be to transmit information, solve problems, deal with general life adjustments, or provide experiences which may change self-concepts, emotional reactions, or teach coping skills.

The size of the group will depend on its function and goals. Work which is very individualized requires a small, intimate group. Themes which are generally relevant can have impact on large numbers.

These approaches fall between group work in a therapeutic setting where the youths have had to acknowledge themselves as patients, with normal activities which are primarily task oriented. The self-developmental and interactional elements of the group activity are considered at least as important as the overt task.

The ways through which changes are achieved may be: information which is fed into the group discussion; the relationships developed and experienced in the group; the group culture which is created and its pressures on members; an examination and understanding of the group interaction; physical, intellectual, and interactional skills which are developed in the group; feedback from persons who share other aspects of daily living; opportunity for role reversal and understanding of others' reactions; increased personal awareness.

Groups provide opportunities for change along the following dimensions. Changes are achieved in the self-image through the individual's taking on a new role and developing a different identity. The individual is seen as different by the members, and new demands are made of him. He learns skills, becomes more competent, and experiences success. His problems and faults as well as his assets are known, and he is accepted as he really is by the leader and the other group members. The individual becomes more sophisticated about human behavior. He learns to observe and understand interactional behavior. He is confronted with his impact on others and is provided with the opportunity to test out different ways of relating to others. He experiences others relating to him in new ways. He can examine what is socially acceptable and why and can learn how community, institution, group, family, and individuals develop and operate and how to increase his social skills. He can reexamine his values and his goals. Groups can provide practice in thinking through and working out problems, in coming to personal and group decisions, and in taking personal and group responsibility.

EDUCATION

There is growing pressure today for the school to take on a socializing role in which youths are prepared to live in the adult world. It is now widely believed that the school should provide a climate in which youth can learn to take increasing responsibility and have a share in decision-making and program-planning. The use of groups is fundamental to this approach whether they are the vehicles for interactive class discussion, parent-faculty-student cooperation, student council government, extracurricular club activities, family life education, or vocational counseling.

Lack of frustration tolerance and motivation for change and learning do not manifest themselves uniformly in the personality. They are intimately connected with the individual's desires and expectations, the opportunities which are offered, and the support which is given. Education offers great opportunities for personal development if the various activities in the school are directed toward the interests of the youth.

The school should be a model for the adult world. If it

is organized as an authoritarian system, it is impossible for youth to learn to take self-responsibility, to make decisions and to function inter- and independently.

Thus, management of the school itself can be used as a means of training children and youth in responsibility and problem-solving if it is organized so that the students participate in the formulation of policy and the maintenance of order. Responsibility is increased as the children advance through school with the classroom being the initial laboratory for leadership training and extending to over-all school functions in the higher grades. Student councils, if they function well, are one example of according responsibility to students. Several experiments are being undertaken in Oregon (Pearl, 1967), where students teach each other and also assist in training teachers, particularly in regard to minority group life styles and the meaning of drugs in the present-day youth culture, through group discussion. In some schools, youth have taken over the management of the cafeteria as a business enterprise.

The formal curriculum can deal with human relations in courses such as human growth and development and family life education; in the examination of human dilemmas and their resolution in an English class; of the way in which the community works in a social science course. Many problems which the children are experiencing elsewhere can be discussed in a less threatening way through analogies to the literature. There is opportunity for consideration of work roles and the management of money in economics classes, not only from the economic framework, but also in terms of the social and psychologic implications of economic independence. Good teaching offers every individual opportunity for success and more self-knowledge and self-mastery through the development of new skills. Homeroom and counseling sessions provide a chance to examine individual and group interactions and goals and to enable the individual to plan for himself and with the group.

A number of writers, such as Jones (1960), have described the use of family life education groups in high school and college as vehicles for personal development on the part of the students. Sheldon Roen (1965) has used an elementary school psychology class as a vehicle for personal development where the children were able to examine the ways they related to each other in the classroom, their feelings, satisfactions, and problems at home, as well as learning about how children grew up.

Lively, interactive classes, in which all students are encouraged to take part and to assist each other in learning can be effective tools for personality development.

Reiff and Riessman (1965) have emphasized the double pay-off of the "Helper Principle," where students, in being trained to tutor and in tutoring others, improve their own performance. Similarly, in Junior Counseling training, the counselors in their training groups learn about human relations. They study themselves in their interactions to each other in seminar groups, and they test out their perceptions and gain more understanding and mastery of themselves in their counseling of others. Two students, for instance, who had great difficulty in tolerating very dependent, demanding, and clinging children, learned much about their own feelings about themselves and their families in examining this problem.

In some school systems, such as in Montgomery County, Maryland, and in the "Street Schools," students have taken the initiative in mobilizing community resources to supplement and expand formal academic study. In some areas, schools have formed a parent-faculty-student group to work together in developing more meaningful curriculum and in the management of school-community relationships (Education Action Teams, Prince George's County, Maryland).

Modern schools not only have to deal with the academic, emotional, and behavioral problems of the students, but they must also find ways to teach them to cope with differences in class, ethnic, and racial life styles. In some schools, interracial student-faculty groups work together to understand and resolve tensions within the school. Another approach is for students to be able to get together with an outside consultant off campus where they can confront each other and can reach beyond the stereotypes and prejudices with which they have grown up. Interracial groups formed around projects and tasks also assist in building new group identifications.

RECREATION

Recreation is indeed a much undervalued opportunity for personality development and change. In an art club, for instance, youths learn not only the mastery of draftsmanship and the use of paint, but also how they perceive the world uniquely, apply themselves, experience emotional and sensory feelings, take interest in each other, make group decisions about program and the allocation of tasks. Dance and drama classes enable youths to be aware of themselves and to be more attuned to their feelings and physical reactions. They provide opportunities for youths to play out different roles and learn how others feel and what their behavior might mean.

In clubs, when youths plan parties, they learn to anticipate problems such as gate crashers and to think through how they will cope with them. They face the fact that the privilege of having parties entails the responsibility for ensuring that they are well-conducted. They promote respect for self and others and the capacity to empathize. They provide opportunities to deal with feelings about authority, rivalry with peers, positive and negative feelings, to understand the ways in which the individual himself manages anxiety and intra-psychic conflict. In examining their own behavior in their group, members can examine how they compete for attention, challenge authority, practice one-upmanship; how they defend against revealing themselves, resist the joys of intimacy because of expected disappointment, rejection, and loss.

Staff at the Bakers Dozen Youth Center in Washington, D.C. (Mitchell et al., 1965), working in a low-income neighborhood, found that many of the children had not learned to deal with problems except through verbal manipulation or violence. Many were deficient in basic skills essential for success in school, such as spatial perception. Because most did not feel they could succeed in the larger society they had adopted an antisocial and delinquent identity. The Center attempted to change the neighborhood climate through the training of youth leaders who ran the recreation groups and served as models for the younger children. It tried to increase the capacity of the youth and children to solve problems in ways which were mutually satisfying, to increase their tolerance of frustration in learning new skills, and to build some educational remediation into the program as well as to enable the children to have fun. In planning trips and parties, the children learned to anticipate and think ahead, to come to group decisions, and to hold responsibly to them. In playing games and in their group interactions, they became conscious of the problems they had in getting along together. They learned to like and trust rather than to exploit each other. Such groups in order to be effective must reach the point of accepting a positive value system so that children recognize, for example, that if they break up a game when they are losing, they are likely to be in trouble or excluded and everyone will have much less fun. The youth and the children both developed physical and intellectual skills which they were able to carry over into their life at home and in school.

In another combined school and recreational program, teenage girls improved their physical coordination and body image through dancing; explored their feelings about parents, boys, and babies while they learned how to cook and sew; and enlarged their perception of the world and their comprehension through trips to Congress, the zoo, art galleries, and science museums (Nash et al., 1967).

In a neighborhood which had a high incidence of teenage out-of-wedlock pregnancy, all the boys and girls participated in a program on the implications of pregnancy which included discussions on biology, family planning, the cost of pregnancy, a variety of ethical approaches. This program was intended to provoke peer-group discussion and resulted in a reevaluation by the teenagers of their behaviors and attitudes to each other. It increased their mutual concern and responsibility and showed a reduction in the number of pregnancies over the following $1\frac{1}{2}$ years (Courvillon, 1967).

EMPLOYMENT

Job counseling and work training have increasingly been seen as valuable opportunities for assisting youth to select careers and to learn how to cope in the world of work. Groups have been used to explore the demands of different work roles. Some group experiences may be directly tied to work tasks as when trainees learn how to cooperate as a team and to relate to their foreman on the job. Other groups form part of training or supervision where youths learn much about themselves as they address themselves to trying out new skills or explore how they have coped with work experiences.

A number of programs have been devised in which different kinds of groups reinforce each other. For example, work experience, skill training, formal education, and residential living may be packaged into a comprehensive program. Although such groups are task-focused and discussion or activities are related to the task, the use of the group to help the individual change and develop himself is of central importance, and the quality of interpersonal experience and discussion is the primary value of these groups. The role of the leader is an active one, and the groups are structured so that the boundaries of the group and the demands on the members are clear. Regression is not stimulated or encouraged through fantasy, and the examination of early memories and unconscious material is avoided.

The Job Corps (1966) has designed an integrated program in which opportunity for personal and social development is provided in a residential job-training setting. The program has four components: formal education, vocational training, group life, and community recreation.

The group-life unit deals with the problems of daily living, works on troubles that start on the job, plans recreation, and considers the aspirations, goals, and problems after the youths leave the program. Because the youths are drawn from many cultural backgrounds, they have to come to terms with differences and recognize that there are many customs, views, and attitudes which, if not adopted, must at least be accepted and tolerated.

Another example was the Howard University New Careers program (MacLennan et al., 1966) which was developed to create opportunities for out-of-school, out-of-work youths from socially disadvantaged backgrounds to enter careers in a variety of human services and to train them for such work. Here, too, the various components of the training were designed to reinforce each other. The program consisted of supervised work in human service which was significant and useful and which could potentially lead to career advancement. This program included skill workshops, remedial education classes, and a core group which served as a medium for social science education and for the kind of counseling described above.

In the workshops, the classes, and particularly in the core group (MacLennan and Klein, 1965), the trainees learned about human relations. They examined the ways in which they dealt with each other and with their clients: children in school, day care, recreation or institutions, adults in hospital. They learned to wonder whether children, when they cry, are tired, hungry, angry, frightened, or trying to get attention. They examined why they themselves reacted differently to different children. They worked on their own values and concepts of themselves. For instance, when one of the trainees was arrested for gambling and arrived late to work, the group members examined the relationship between private life and work and to what extent they could and should be models for the children. They first thought that each person's private life was his own. Then they began to consider how, by being arrested, the aide might have let the children down or been fired himself. Finally, they tackled the problem of how they wanted the children and the parents to think of them, what kind of model they should be. Boys and girls who had resisted education for years began to feel the need to be able to write and speak well, and they began to demand more formal education. They became aware how, when they were uncomfortable, they would start to fight, talk about something else, burst into physical activity, or withdraw into sleep or sullen silence. As they were held to and mastered activities and gained the respect and affection of supervisors and clients, they ceased to see themselves as failures and ne'er-do-wells. Boys and girls with long histories of impulsive or aggressive behavior began to buckle down and to work responsibly and sensitively in this program. Many neighborhood youth corps programs have followed this pattern (MacLennan, 1966).

In many of the poverty programs, youth and other indigenous workers have been employed as research informants and program evaluators because of the specialized knowledge which they possess of their own communities (Grant, et al., 1966). In such activity, they inevitably gain a greater understanding of themselves and the world in which they live, their values and promises, their relationships to others, the way in which they differ from others in their community, the power and structure of their community, and how it fits into the larger society.

CHURCH ACTIVITIES

Organized religion still provides moral leadership for many teenagers; and church groups, whether they are established for social, educational, counseling activities, or philosophical discussion, offer many opportunities for the teenager to learn more about himself, review his values, and develop relationships with peers and adults. Many churches today run groups on human relations and sex education, premarital counseling, prejudice and poverty; and clergy, congregation, and youth join in searching for new roles in modern society.

THE YOUTH MOVEMENTS

No discussion of groups for teenagers as part of normal living could be complete today without at least a brief examination of the groups which are formed by youth themselves as part of their struggle to deal with the problems of the modern world. Some of these, such as the Civil Rights Movement, the student revolution, the environmental protest, are concerned with the reform of adult society. Others are attempts to break away and to experiment with a new way of living or to form a separate society. These include the communes, the runaway pads, the addict groups, the black separatists, and teenage delinquent gangs. All have in common a rejection of the world as it is and a despair that any change can occur through normal democratic means. Still others are attempts by youths to deal by themselves with their own problems, where existing methods are used by peers in the belief that teenagers have better understanding of teenage problems.

Teen businesses, free schools, teen patrols, discotheques, hot lines, and youth-managed counseling services offer youth prototypes of adult institutions run by youth. Many of these efforts are stimulated and encouraged by young adults who act as resource persons, mediators, and facilitators, providing liaison between youths and adults. It is remarkable that most of the youths who take part in one or another of these movements, unless they become too physically damaged or stigmatized or locked out by society, settle down to perform the normal tasks of adult life once the adolescent crisis is over. These efforts exemplify, in enlarged form, the normal process of adolescence: the rejection of adult values, the separation and dissociation from adults, the defiance of authority, the search for new experiences, the struggle for identity and significance, the need to experiment. Many of these movements attract the brightest and most mature of modern youth. The most extreme are sometimes led by the most disturbed, who find an outlet for their upset in a significant cause but who have difficulty in perceiving the boundaries and limits of reality.

PROCESS AND MANEUVERS IN GROUPS OF ADOLESCENTS

Whatever type of group is planned, it is important to recognize that there is a uniform process in all groups and that the leaders need to be aware of the underlying emotional dynamics. All groups follow the same sequence. Members become acquainted, identify a common purpose, test each other and the leader in order to develop a degree of trust, establish a way of working together, struggle to conduct their business, and ultimately disband. Each phase poses its own problems and arouses particular feelings: anxiety at starting; competition for position; pride in successful resolution of problems; sadness at parting (MacLennan, 1968, and MacLennan and Felsenfeld, 1970).

The leader is crucial to all groups for, in one way or another, he teaches the members how to work together. In teenage groups particularly, the leader must be free enough to allow the youngsters to take increasing responsibility for the group, yet firm enough not to be overrun and defeated. Although youngsters often try to depose the leader, in their hearts they do not wish to succeed, for a weak leader is no good to them. Testing operations are an inevitable aspect of the early stages of groups since members seek to know where they stand in the group and whether they can trust each other and the leader. These testing operations include griping against authority, complaining and blaming others, attacking the leader verbally either directly or indirectly, seeing whether the leader will permit things which they know are against the rules, and trying to see whether he will betray them. Members want to know what the leader is like as a person and what he stands for. The leader is expected to make his values clear even if they are not always agreeable to the youth. However, the acceptance of differences while maintaining the relationship is often an important new experience for the youth. Task-oriented groups reduce the pressures of testing, but they still continue even if in more subtle ways.

When the group is first formed, members are very concerned about whether the group will be effective. Loss of a member is seen as a potential threat to the group; and when others are absent or late, members are afraid that they are being rejected or that the group will dissolve.

Anxiety is high in all adolescent groups; and members,

particularly those in their early teens, may well use physical activity as a means of tension release. Boys and girls touch each other, wrestle, giggle, get up and move around. The leader is faced with the task of judging how much of this to permit and when it becomes a resistance and should be stopped. Some leaders use activity to reduce anxiety. Anxiety-provoking silences are also hard for youth to tolerate and should not be allowed to go on too long. In general, the leader tends to be more active in teenage than in adult groups.

Once the members have become more comfortable with each other, they are able to express their feelings and opinions more freely, to confront differences, and to express their intimate anxieties. However, resistance to self-revelation, learning, and change is an integral part of all therapeutic work; and in all groups which involve the verbal discussion of experiences, behavior, feelings, or problems, leaders will find both individual and group resistances. Members avoid involvement through silence or chatter, through diverting discussion from important issues, or through dwelling unduly on inconsequential detail. Some members repeatedly bring up issues but then refuse to deal with them. Others agree without agreeing. Still others monopolize the conversation or talk so vaguely that no one can understand what they are saying. Boasting is a frequent sign of uneasiness early in the group. The leader's function is to understand the underlying concern and help the group to respond appropriately. If a group member is allowed to continue to resist for long, it usually indicates that his activities have a function for other members in the group. Members often enter into collusion to avoid working on the tasks of the group. They will resist through mutual admiration, through fighting, or through joining in diversionary activities. Sometimes they will allow a member to monopolize the group's attention for it keeps the heat off them, or perhaps they may scapegoat a member and thus redirect their anger from themselves or the leader to a safer target. In moments of great anxiety, the group will often unite in an attempt to place all responsibility on to the leader and will assault him with dependent demands. It is important for the leader to understand what is going on so that he can react appropriately, for the same behavior in different contexts can have very different meanings. He must decide whether to tackle the group or the individual, to explore, confront, divert, or ignore.

Competition goes on constantly in adolescent groups with and for the leader. Members compare themselves with each other and deal with the struggle in their own customary ways. Some play the role of the sick or the weak or the isolated. Others work very hard, compete by being good or by attention-getting, disruptive behavior; others still by playing dumb. All, however, want to be loved, cared about, to care and to be respected. These roles which people have learned to play from early childhood in their own families manifest themselves in all kinds of groups and, if dysfunctional, must be dealt with in one way or another. Sometimes, it is enough for the leader and the group to support some behaviors and ignore others. Sometimes, however, the misbehaving teenager may be so persistent and disruptive that he must be confronted directly and helped to understand how he is defeating himself. Whatever the leader chooses to do, his concern for the individual and the group must be both visible and genuine.

Adolescents can often be very difficult as well as great to work with, for their feelings are intense and their anxiety contagious. The leader may have a hard time avoiding getting caught up in these feelings. If members find that the leader does not seem to understand them or to care, they easily become impatient and angry. Their demands on adults are as great as their inner condemnations of themselves. Leaders have to be free enough to respond to the group's concerns. For instance, if a group wishes to talk about sexual matters and the leader cannot face this, he will seem unresponsive to the member's concerns, and they are likely to attack him or to withdraw from the group in disgust.

Groups of young teenagers are more volatile than those of 16- to 19-year-olds. The youngsters have a hard time staying with problems and difficulties and respond better to positive approaches and opportunities to experience success. Leaders can, however, by following the themes of the group interaction (the underlying, unstated concerns about separation, inadequacy, loneliness, etc.), respond by word or action to clarify, confront, confirm, or reassure.

The termination of a group, even if it has only been of short duration, will have significance for its members. There will be feelings of loss mingled with relief or satisfaction and attempts to deal with unhappiness. Sometimes group members ignore the fact that the group is about to end and work as if the group continuing forever. Other times they relive the history of the group or make plans for renewed meetings to soften the blow of parting. Groups, like individuals, may regress into earlier, more dependent behavior. Also individual members deal with loss differently. Some leave very abruptly, others deny all caring, while others may express their feelings openly. If some are able to advance successfully or "graduate" from the group before others, all the members may have very mixed feelings. The successful member is likely to be both glad and a little guilty. The others who are left behind may feel jealous, glad, and sorry. Leaders too may have loved the group and find it hard to let it end. However, endings are also beginnings; and when members leave the group, they are going on to new opportunities. The group experience is a part of each member's life and can never be taken away. The leader's task is to enable himself and the

members to deal with feelings, separate, and move hopefully into the future.

ISSUES RAISED BY THESE APPROACHES

There are several issues which have to be dealt with
when management and resolution of psychologic problems
are considered as an integral part of everyday living. Trial
and error must be accepted as the norm rather than
perfection and the youths allowed to learn from their
mistakes. Adults need to be able to turn over part of the
responsibility to the youths and to relinquish some control
over what happens without too much anxiety. Too often
when a problem occurs, adults take back the leadership
which they had given up instead of allowing the youths to
work on the problem. Instead, the climate should favor a
striving for greater maturity and improved functioning.
This emphasis requires a reorganization of staff roles.
Training is usually required for administrators to learn
how to develop a positive milieu and for line staff to
understand and manage individuals and groups in dynamic
interaction.

Because interventions occur as part of daily life, it
may not always be possible to select group members as
carefully as one would wish. Leaders, therefore, need to be
alert to any adverse reactions on the part of individuals
who may require some special help. While groups and
activities are not presented as treatment, there should be
an understanding that one function is to assist participants
to learn more about themselves and others, and to increase
their capacity to function effectively. Youths are expected
to try to deal honestly with situations which arise and to
assist each other in solving problems. It is no longer
regarded as valid for members to conspire or to hide
problems from the group.

This also necessitates a change in the attitudes and

relationships of the interveners, be they trainers, counselors, teachers, or senior colleagues, to each other and to the youths. The interveners have to be willing to submit their own opinions and actions to scrutiny and to recognize and admit that they do not know all the answers. The dichotomous system between authorities and the rest with its divided loyalties and secrets and miscommunications so well described by Goffman (1961) and illustrated by Empey (1966) and Polsky (1962) is reduced to a single interacting group in which all attempt to achieve, in task-related fashion, improved functioning and and common goals.

When self-development and therapy become a part of normal groups, the leaders are required to be more knowledgeable about individuals, groups, and institutions. Whether they are teachers, recreation group leaders, supervisors, administrators, or clergymen, they need to be able to recognize the meaning of individual and group behavior, to understand that individuals are affected by group and institutional pressures, and to be more aware of their own reactions. Leaders of all groups require some skill in group management. Groups which are designed to create anxiety and conflict in the service of change and which operate in a climate of emotionality and tension must have leaders who are trained and competent to deal with the dynamic pressures which are aroused.

This implies a need for change in the preparation of personnel who deal with youth and creates a new relationship with the mental health specialists who now must play major roles as educators, trainers, consultants. Mental helath specialists may also become teachers or job trainers or recreation workers in the management of some groups. The selection of those who work with youth requires careful consideration. People who are threatened by the impulsiveness, aggressiveness, and demands of youth and who respond by repressiveness, tightening controls, or rejection are not suitable to assist in the psychosocial development of youth.

These approaches raise questions about whether all problems can and should be worked on within normal settings or whether some youths, because of the severity of their problems, must have a specially designed therapeutic environment. It has been found that some violent and very difficult youths have been able to respond remarkably and give up their irresponsibility and lack of self-control when placed in a situation where expectations and opportunities were congruent and positive and where the environment reinforced the group experience. Some repetitive and aggressive offenders, who had spent years in delinquent training schools, have been able to learn and to accept responsible positions in New Careers Programs (MacLennan et al., 1966). Beyond restructuring the environment, it may only be necessary to provide facilities such as the hot lines and free clinics where upset teenagers can find assistance in crisis and support in their search for significance and respect.

Perhaps, too, the greatest effort has to be expended on adults to assist them to be able to accept and enjoy the struggles of youth. If adults could recognize the needs of youth to separate, to innovate, and to make a place for themselves; if they could support when appropriate and defend their own rights without guilt, the generation gap might seem a less formidable obstacle in Western society and youth might mature with less trauma and upset.

REFERENCES

Courvillon, B. S. (1967): Preventing Premature Pregnancies. Research Proposal to the Office of Economic Opportunity and the Ford Foundation for Family Life Association of Metropolitan Washington, Inc.

Empey, L. T. (1966): A Social Systems Approach for Working in Small Groups with Socially Deprived Youth. Presented at American

Group Psychotherapy Association Annual Conference, Philadelphia, Pa.

Goffman, E. (1961): *Asylums*. Anchor Books, Doubleday, New York.

Goffman, E. (1963): *Stigma; Notes on the Management of Spoiled Identity*. Prentice-Hall, Englewood Cliffs, N. J.; p. 147.

Grant, J. D., et al. (1966): The Offender as a Correctional Manpower Resource: Its Implementation. Institute for the Study of Crime and Delinquency, NIMH, Asilomar, Calif.

Jones, R. (1960): *An Application of Psychoanalysis to Education*. Charles C Thomas Springfield, Ill., p. 134.

MacLennan, B. W. (1968): Group approaches to the problems of socially deprived youth: The classical psychotherapeutic model. Int. J. Group Psychother. 18(4):481–494.

MacLennan, B. W., and Felsenfeld, N. (1968 [paperback, 1970]): *Group Counseling and Psychotherapy with Adolescents*. Columbia University Press, New York.

MacLennan, B. W., and Klein, W. L. (1965): Utilization of groups in job training for the socially deprived. Int. J. Group Psychother., 15(4):424–433.

MacLennan, B. W., et al. (1966): Training for new careers. Community Mental Health Journal 2(2): 135–141.

Mitchell, L. E., et al. (1965): *A Mobile Therapeutic Community for Adolescents*. Howard University Center for Youth and Community Studies, Washington, D. C.

Nast, E. L., et al. (March 1967): A Collaborative School-Mental Health Program for Disadvantaged Teenagers. Presented at 44th Annual Meeting of the American Orthopsychiatric Association, Washington, D. C., p. 15.

Pearl, A. (1967): Training for responsible citizenship in the school. (Personal communication.)

Polsky, H. W. (1962): *Cottage Six*. Russell Sage Foundation, New York.

Prince George's County Board of Education Report (mimeo.) (1970): Education Action Teams, Upper Marlboro, Maryland.

Reiff, R., and Riessman, F. (1965): The indigenous nonprofessional. Community Mental Health Journal, Monograph Series, No. 1.

Roen, S. (1965): Primary Prevention in the Classroom through a Teaching Program in the Behavioral Sciences. University of Rochester Conference on Emergent Approaches to Mental Health Problems.

The Job Corps, A Dialogue (1966): American Child, Vol. 48 (whole issue).

Chapter 15

STREET WORK PROGRAM WITH YOUTH

Rix G. Rogers

An immediate question that can be raised is why the need for street work? The answer stems from the fact that many of society's institutions remain aloof from the people they are supposed to serve. Although this has always been a problem for some people (notably persons in poverty and many newcomers to the country), the phenomenon now seems much more widespread among the youth sector.

Currently, there are on the streets many young people with serious social handicaps, in addition to other physical and emotional problems which are more familiar. Many youths are having great difficulty in experiencing meaningful interpersonal relationships with their peers, as well as with adults.

Such social alienation is aggravated by the lack of a central and gripping goal orientation for our society. A society with a sense of direction seems to foster a sense of security among the dependent persons; however, during times of ambiguity and diversity in society the dependent person can easily find himself alone, fearful and apathetic.

Indigenous staff have repeatedly demonstrated their ability to build relationships and this, coupled with the expertise of the professional community, presents a new and essential partnership pattern for reaching and dealing with alienation.

Dr. John Unwin, referring to the Canadian scene, notes: "Particularly since the summer――――, when large numbers of rootless North American Youth converged on Canadian cities, professionals in a number of disciplines have noted, in a good number of these adolescents and young adults, certain types of behavior styles of relating and qualities of mood which, it is here proposed, constitute a syndrome of depressive reaction." (Unwin, 1969.)

From our experience gained in the last 3 years we consider it essential for communities to develop four major service capabilities for a comprehensive approach in local sectors. This service system should be made up of all the organizations and groups that have resources and expertise which can be mobilized. These can be described briefly as:

1. **Contact Capability**

   An outreach activity utilizing street workers to contact youth who tend to avoid institutions of any kind. This involves developing relationships with the whole range of youth and their problems. The contact system developed in Montreal by the YMCA is now in its fourth year of operation.

2. **Crisis Intervention Capability**

   This is characterized by emergency telephone-answering services 24 hours a day, walk-in youth clinics, and professional resource persons on call, as well as out-patient clinics of hospitals. To a degree some "drop-in centers" also provide crisis counseling services.

3. **Alternative Programs**

These are activities which stimulate constructive alternatives to youth alienation, hard-core drug abuse, and acts of hostility. Examples are encounter groups, special employment projects, and projects like media workshops. Drop-in centers designed as social therapeutic communities are an important resource in working with apathy and negativism.

4. **Special Institutional Services**

Local teaching hospitals, sensitive to changing community needs and supporting local youth clinics, represent a most essential service. Other community institutions, including a wide range of government services, can provide particular functions as required.

It is obvious that much must be done in a comprehensive way to deal with the problems of youth alienation. Even the hospital, which we tend to look to as the major institution for treating medical and psychiatric problems, is presently limited to a serious degree. There is not an adequate system of support services in the community to work with the youth in difficulty, both before he gets to the hospital, and after he is ready to leave.

THE CONCEPT OF STREET WORK

The concept of street work is the attempt of young workers to reach young people in their milieu, to assist them as they try to develop meaningful ways of relating to themselves, to their environment, to their peers and to society. This work is sometimes also called "detached youth work," but for the purposes of this discussion will be called street work.

Much of the workers' time is spent on the street, directly involved with the mobile patterns of young people. The workers use their time seeking out and making contact with young people in their own surroundings, whether it be in a park, restaurant, or drop-in center. Many of these young people are hard-to-reach or alienated youth. For a variety of reasons they are distrustful of society in general and extremely reluctant to participate in the on-going structured programs of youth-serving organizations or to use the available medical services of local hospitals. There are usually four phases that the workers go through to establish rapport with alienated individuals:

1. The contact phase . . . getting out into the milieu and contacting people where they are located.
2. Rapport building with individuals and developing a sound relationship with them.
3. Short-range need satisfaction . . . characterized by medical needs, shelter, clothing, food, etc. In this phase attempts are made to direct individuals to the resources that can provide for these short-range needs. If the resources aren't available, attempts are made to get the individuals to organize themselves to help satisfy their own needs.
4. Long-range need satisfaction . . . characterized by extensive counselling program, activities that help change environments, getting back into education programs, job retraining programs, etc. (Detached Work Unit, 1969, p. 3.)

In essence the street worker is a "catalyst" with several dimensions. Diagrammatically these can be viewed as involving:

a. One-to-one relationships,
    ↓
b. One-to-a-small group,
    ↓
c. To the small group, plus various resources in the community required to meet needs,
    ↓
d. To various institutions and their operators and to new areas of activity.

The street work approach has evolved over the last 20 years and is now utilized in most large cities in North America by established youth-serving organizations as well as by indigenous groups and associations. In the Montreal YMCA the following are the stated goals of the street work program:

1. To help youth identify their problems and/or concerns.
2. To confront youth with the need to solve their problems and/or concerns which are detrimental to themselves or the community.
3. To muster community resources to meet the needs of the individuals' problems or concerns and, where those resources are irrelevant or non-existent, to change or create new services.
4. To involve youth in a caring relationship with adults, including family relationships and other adults in the community. (Detached Work Unit, 1969, p. 1.)

Philosophy of Indigenous Involvement

The development of special services such as drop-in centers or youth clinics must involve the indigenous population in the designing of the organization and in the implementation of the service or activity. This is a fundamental concept. Such an approach ensures that the service "belongs" to the group it is serving. This pattern also ensures continuous feedback about the value of the service and has become an important measure in assessing the value of any particular service.

THE CONCEPT IN OPERATION

Team Development

We consider it highly desirable to develop street work teams, rather than have a worker completely on his own. The strains of this emotionally demanding work are eased by maintaining close contact with colleagues on a day-to-day basis. The team should comprise two or three full-time workers, augmented with part-time paid workers and volunteers when appropriate and when available.

Continuity

Experience suggests that it is also highly desirable to maintain a street work project on a year-round basis and for a cycle of 3 years, if at all possible. Under these conditions the team can be augmented during the summer months or at any other crucial period without disrupting continuity. Full-time team workers must be given time to develop relationships and follow through on individual problems or group projects which may emerge. This has implications for funding, and for long-range planning on the part of the initiating group.

On a regular basis, particularly at the end of a 2- or 3-year cycle, a careful assessment of each project can help determine whether the work in that community should be continued, expanded, reduced, or altered. Specific targets can be set regarding the solution of various problems.

Selection and Qualifications of Workers

This is perhaps the most crucial factor in developing an effective and constructive service. Experience over the past 5 years in the Montreal YMCA suggests that many of the usual measures of competency—such as formal education and previous experience—are not in themselves adequate. The following seem to be the most important factors:

1. **Empathy**

   The potential worker must exhibit a high degree of empathy towards disadvantaged, or hard-to-reach young people. He or she must have the ability to accept other individuals, even though they may not like some of their behavior.

2. **Emotional Stability, Inner Strength and Ability to Cope**
    Since the worker will face an intensely emotional environment in his day-to-day work, he must have the ability to cope effectively with strong emotions, and not become immobilized by them. Often, personal hostility will be vented towards the worker in the beginning stages of developing relationships. The capacity to deal with it, without suffering excessive anxiety and depression, is essential.

3. **Integrity, Personal Values and Commitment**
    As the worker functions in the community he brings himself as the principal resource in his daily work. His principles, his values and his discretion are constantly being tested and challenged.

    The worker must have a firm sense of his own values and goals in life and understand his own motivation for the work he is doing. He must also resolve the relationship of his own personal goals to those of his organization. If he cannot feel that these are compatible, he will be hindered in the forthrightness of his own stance and commitment.

4. **Emotional Capacity and Awareness of Feelings**
    In addition to his rational powers to solve problems and exercise sound judgment, the worker must have great capacity to relate sympathetically to people around him. This is the prime basis for developing trust.

    One of the major lacks in the lives of many young people is the lack of ability of many adults to relate to them on an emotional basis. Many hard-to-reach youth, in turn, have lost their capacity to feel and to be spontaneous. This problem is central in the activity of the street worker.

5. **Interdependent Qualities of Relationships, Personal Maturity**

An important function of the worker is to provide a link between individual young people and the community. An essential qualification of this role is the ability to make use of available community resources. This calls for ability to relate to a variety of organizations.

Personal maturity in coping with imperfect services and moderate resources is required if excessive frustration and counterdependent feelings are to be managed.

In addition, while the value of the street worker is becoming increasingly apparent, there are still a number of professionals and members of organizations in the community who are not entirely convinced. The individual worker must be prepared to devote time and energy to establishing his credibility.

The preceding criteria are considered most important. Knowledge and training in the fields of psychology, sociology, anthropology, political science, or social work are plus factors.

The age of most workers is between 19 and 25 years. In many cases it is preferable that the majority of them be of legal age (21 years), but this is not essential.

Female workers can be just as competent as males, depending on the milieu and the geographic setting. Workers in the inner-city, especially in gang areas, tend to be male. In other sectors, female workers have proved just as effective as their male counterparts.

Orientation and Training Programs

It is essential that adequate time be taken during the initial stages of employment to discuss and debate the goals of the program and the nature of the employing organization. For newcomers, meetings with other experienced workers can help develop confidence. In the launching of a new project, it is beneficial if one of the team members has experience in the field.

Close supportive relationships with the back-up support system (see next section) of the organization provides an in-service training dimension which seems to contribute most to individual worker's learning, growth, and competence. This framework also helps the targets for the project. These, in turn, become the criteria for assessing progress and results.

Normal targets usually encompass such factors as unusual apathy, drug abuse problems, lack of needed services in the community, excessive hostility towards the community, serious unemployment problems, and family difficulties.

Two other training patterns have been found extremely valuable by the Montreal YMCA street work unit:
1. A weekly community meeting of all workers, including indigenous workers from the other projects in the community.

    The chance to meet weekly helps build rapport and fosters among workers across the city a feeling of belonging to a special community of their own. Beefs, tensions, and anxieties can be aired. This provides feedback for everybody concerned, and allows for a venting of pent-up feelings. Administrative problems, or hang-ups with the organization, can also be identified regularly and resolved before they reach crisis proportions. If there is an over-all community problem developing, it can be identified and tackled in a concerted manner.

The development of interrelationships helps with communication flow, and provides an over-all picture of the work going on in the city. Above all, the community meeting helps to offset a sense of isolation and loneliness for workers in any sector of the city.

2. Periodically (e.g., 3-month intervals) for the total street work group to move away from their milieu for a week-end training experience in another setting (preferably a somewhat isolated residential training center). On these occasions, special resource people from the psychiatric, legal, or community development fields can be utilized to probe, in greater depth, some of the special factors being dealt with on the street.

Since this is a relatively new field of work, greater insight also may be gained about the general nature of this approach and the special dynamics which seem to be involved.

Back-up Support Services of the Street Work Program

After 4 years of street work and the development of several project teams, it has become evident that a large program, to be effective, requires a very competent back-up leadership team. The following are some of the major functions required:
1. Worker selection, orientation and placement.
2. Continuous involvement with workers in the field, monitoring developing problems, responding to emergency needs of staff, and involvement in the assessment process in the projects.
3. Administrative functions related to budgeting, payroll, etc., and helping to secure special funds.

4. Interpretative and educational functions. The support team is the prime vehicle for linking street work projects to the rest of the organization, and to the community, and working on the needs of integrating these innovative services as part of the organization. There is an external function of data collection, sharing and interpretation with all pertinent professionals, community institutions, and various governmental bodies, in the whole field of youth in difficulty.

5. General leadership and initiative for meeting gaps in service, developing new projects, relating to a wide variety of other community indigenous activity, and operating a wide variety of special services which are integral to the street work activity. Such special items include leadership for encounter groups, sensitivity-training events, operational support for walk-in youth clinics, and pilot projects such as media workshops.

Regional Coordination

Along with street work activity in any given region, it is now considered necessary to have some full-time staff member assume the role of "resources and information coordinator." In most cases this person is not a street worker, but another designated staff person either from the YMCA or some other agency.

The task assigned is to develop and maintain effective liaison with all potential resources in that community and to work closely with street workers to utilize these resources. Through this approach, strenuous efforts are being made to develop more effective communication among agencies, hospitals, professional personnel, and governmental services.

Voluntary groups, service clubs, and home and school associations are all being involved in discussions of local problems and needs. In one community (City of Verdun) the street work activity and related services are now jointly sponsored by all of these community organizations.

The total mobilization of community resources and the effective collaboration of professional workers, along with indigenous personnel, is the goal of this approach. What is required is a network of services in the community including contact capability, crisis intervention capability, alternative programs, and special institutional services.

We have found that ineffectiveness in part of this network seriously limits the effectiveness of the others; hence, the need for collaboration and mutual planning regarding services for alienated youth.

BENEFITS OF A STREET WORK PROGRAM

From our experience to date we believe that the following benefits can be noted regarding the street work program:

1. A street work program provides early access to youth in trouble who would not be served until their problems became major crises, if it were not for this outreach approach.
2. The program through first-hand relationships at a grass-roots level with hard-to-reach young people provides pertinent data about the ideas, problems and concerns of youth as they develop in the community. These are essential data for the community to better understand the perceptions of youth today.
3. The program provides an opportunity for dialogue with "disenchanted" young people, and to influence and to be influenced by their feelings, attitudes and perceptions.
4. Valuable feedback is gained about the effectiveness of present services to youth, and about new needs which are unmet. These are essential data for good

planning by the various organizations and for the reshaping of organizations where required.

5. There are some indications that street work is an integrating force, helping to bridge the gaps between alienated youth and the general community. There are very few of these "integrating" or "connecting" forces in today's society and yet they seem desperately needed.

6. It has been our experience that a trust relationship developed between a worker and an individual can be readily and quickly transferrable to a competent and empathetic professional in the community, when it has been determined that professional help is needed. The street worker, then, is a means of helping to utilize to a much higher degree the many resources that exist in our society, but that are not fully utilized.

7. Another value of the street worker to the professional community and to youth-serving institutions is an immediate feedback mechanism regarding the inadequacies or gaps in existing services. The "blind spots" which often exist in the professional community can be corrected continuously if the beedback is accepted and utilized.

CRITERIA FOR ASSESSMENT

The assessment question is particularly important since street work involves a relatively new methodology and because so much of the measurement of the work now done is based on a subjective judgment.

While a good deal of assessment will continue to be subjective, it is also important that some objective measures be made as well. Currently, in the Montreal program, research is under way in the field of worker recruitment, selection, and training, and the relationship of street work to levels of juvenile delinquency in the inner-city.

Objective research should be part of any street work program, since it is only through this process that ultimate measures and conclusions can be verified. The number of youths that a worker can be expected to influence is difficult to determine precisely. Experience so far suggests that an established worker may have intensive relationships with 50 or more individuals, casual relationships with up to 300, and may be known by reputation in the area by some 700 youths. Where a drop-in center is an integral part of the workers' activity, a team may have considerable influence with 2000 or 3000 youths.

One measure which is looked at closely is the change cycle of a worker in his intensive relationships. There should be a continuing change in this constituency over a 3-month period. If there is not, there may be an indication of strong fixed dependency on the worker.

The goal is to help the individual move beyond a stage of dependency on the worker; to take more and more initiative in expanding his interpersonal relationships with others. Continuing analysis and discussions with the street work support staff are one means of monitoring this progress, along with the other established targets for the project team. Perhaps the most important factor in assessing the progress of street work is direct feedback from the youth themselves. Integral to this field of work is the assimilation of a constant flow of data from the street. These have been essential data in monitoring progress of the work.

OPERATION PROBLEMS

Credibility and Acceptance of This Work by the Community

Tensions are inevitably created within the sponsoring organization and continuing energy is required to work on these various dynamics all the time. Some professionals still hold to the view that no one but a highly trained professional has a legitimate place in working with troubled individuals.

Integrating the efforts of the indigenous worker with the many professionals in the community is also difficult. The notion that each can make a significant contribution to an over-all community problem is not yet readily accepted.

Evaluation

The fact that assessment remains highly subjective, makes it difficult to provide objective evidence for this new field of work.

Hostility, Counterdependent Behavior and the Problems of Militancy

Workers and their organizations must be able to distinguish between a variety of principled activists on the one hand, and subversives on the other. Workers find themselves in the midst of racial conflict, the new left, radicalism, and the drug scene.

At some points workers will come close to organized crime and may be personally threatened. All of these dynamics go along with intensive involvement. Workers, as they get closer to youth and gain insight into urgent problems, become impatient with the rate of change in the community, and in various organizations. The continuing lag between "need" and "need response" tends to be a constant source of frustration for people in the field.

Goals

It tends to be assumed by most professionals that the treatment of the individual involves helping him to adjust to society. In fact, society must change too, and the new goal problem is to help both the individual and society to change in appropriate ways.

As the street work program becomes deeply involved with "gut" issues in the neighborhood, continuing clarification is required by all concerned regarding the end results everyone is working for.

Financing

A comprehensive street work program is costly and does not produce operational income. In addition to the cost of the workers on the street, the back-up support system is an added expense. In Montreal, several municipal governments are supporting programs in their areas. Foundation grants and individual donations have also provided help. In the long term, more substantial governmental funding will be required if this new field of work is to be continued.

Lack of Collaboration

Most community organizations and institutions operate quite independently and, although cordial relationships may exist, there has been little collaborative effort in the past. The development of growing alienation among young people calls for an integrated effort by a variety of organizations. We have experienced some hopeful beginnings, but much more must be done before there is truly an overall community approach to the problem.

REFERENCES

Detached Work Unit, Montreal YMCA (August 1969): Unit Description. Montreal.

Unwin, J. R. (1969): Depression in Alienated Youth. Paper presented at the 19th Annual Meeting of the Canadian Psychiatric Association, Toronto, Ontario, June 12.

DATE DUE

DEC 1 0 1973			
DEC 11 1973			
APR 2 7 1982			
APR 7 1982			
APR 2 7 1987			
APR 1 1989			
GAYLORD			PRINTED IN U.S.A.

YOUTH:

Problems and Approaches